DELIBERATE PRACTICE IN
ACCELERATED EXPERIENTIAL DYNAMIC PSYCHOTHERAPY

Essentials of Deliberate Practice Series
Tony Rousmaniere and Alexandre Vaz, Series Editors

Deliberate Practice in Accelerated Experiential Dynamic Psychotherapy
Natasha C. N. Prenn, Hanna Levenson, Alexandre Vaz, and Tony Rousmaniere

Deliberate Practice in Career Counseling
Jennifer M. Taylor, Alexandre Vaz, and Tony Rousmaniere

Deliberate Practice in Child and Adolescent Psychotherapy
Jordan Bate, Tracy A. Prout, Tony Rousmaniere, and Alexandre Vaz

Deliberate Practice in Cognitive Behavioral Therapy
James F. Boswell and Michael J. Constantino

Deliberate Practice in Dialectical Behavior Therapy
Tali Boritz, Shelley McMain, Alexandre Vaz, and Tony Rousmaniere

Deliberate Practice in Emotion-Focused Therapy
Rhonda N. Goldman, Alexandre Vaz, and Tony Rousmaniere

Deliberate Practice in Emotionally Focused Couple Therapy
Hanna Levenson, Sam Jinich, Alexandre Vaz, and Tony Rousmaniere

Deliberate Practice in Interpersonal Psychotherapy
Olga Belik, Scott Fairhurst, Jessica M. Schultz, Scott Stuart, Alexandre Vaz, and Tony Rousmaniere

Deliberate Practice in Motivational Interviewing
Jennifer K. Manuel, Denise Ernst, Alexandre Vaz, and Tony Rousmaniere

Deliberate Practice in Multicultural Therapy
Jordan Harris, Joel Jin, Sophia Hoffman, Selina Phan, Tracy A. Prout, Tony Rousmaniere, and Alexandre Vaz

Deliberate Practice in Psychedelic-Assisted Therapy
Shannon Dames, Andrew Penn, Monnica Williams, Joseph A. Zamaria, Tony Rousmaniere, and Alexandre Vaz

Deliberate Practice in Psychodynamic Psychotherapy
Hanna Levenson, Volney Gay, and Jeffrey L. Binder

Deliberate Practice in Rational Emotive Behavior Therapy
Mark D. Terjesen, Kristene A. Doyle, Raymond A. DiGiuseppe, Alexandre Vaz, and Tony Rousmaniere

Deliberate Practice in Schema Therapy
Wendy T. Behary, Joan M. Farrell, Alexandre Vaz, and Tony Rousmaniere

Deliberate Practice in Systemic Family Therapy
Adrian J. Blow, Ryan B. Seedall, Debra L. Miller, Tony Rousmaniere, and Alexandre Vaz

ESSENTIALS OF DELIBERATE PRACTICE SERIES

TONY ROUSMANIERE AND ALEXANDRE VAZ, SERIES EDITORS

DELIBERATE PRACTICE IN
ACCELERATED EXPERIENTIAL DYNAMIC PSYCHOTHERAPY

NATASHA C. N. PRENN

HANNA LEVENSON

ALEXANDRE VAZ

TONY ROUSMANIERE

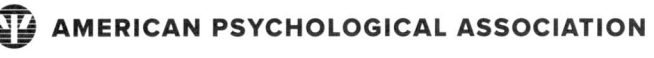 AMERICAN PSYCHOLOGICAL ASSOCIATION

Published by
American Psychological Association
750 First Street, NE
Washington, DC 20002
https://www.apa.org

Order Department
https://www.apa.org/pubs/books
order@apa.org

Typeset in Cera Pro by Circle Graphics, Inc., Reisterstown, MD

Printer: Sheridan Books, Chelsea, MI
Cover Designer: Mark Karis

Library of Congress Cataloging-in-Publication Data

Names: Prenn, Natasha C. N., author. | Levenson, Hanna, 1945- author. |
    Vaz, Alexandre, author. | Rousmaniere, Tony, author. | American
    Psychological Association, publisher.
Title: Deliberate practice in accelerated experiential dynamic
    psychotherapy / by Natasha C. N. Prenn, Hanna Levenson, Alexandre Vaz,
    and Tony Rousmaniere.
Other titles: Essentials of deliberate practice series
Description: Washington, DC : American Psychological Association, [2025] |
    Series: Essentials of deliberate practice series | Includes
    bibliographical references and index.
Identifiers: LCCN 2024032466 (print) | LCCN 2024032467 (ebook) | ISBN
    9781433842900 (paperback) | ISBN 9781433842917 (ebook)
Subjects: MESH: Psychotherapy--education | Psychotherapy--methods | Role
    Playing | Problems and Exercises | BISAC: PSYCHOLOGY / Education &
    Training | PSYCHOLOGY / Clinical Psychology
Classification: LCC RC480.5 (print) | LCC RC480.5 (ebook) | NLM WM 18.2
    | DDC 616.89/14--dc23/eng/20241203
LC record available at https://lccn.loc.gov/2024032466
LC ebook record available at https://lccn.loc.gov/2024032467

https://doi.org/10.1037/0000439-000

Printed in the United States of America

10 9 8 7 6 5 4 3 2

To Hanna and Alex

—Natasha Prenn

To Avis and Donna, my "chosen sisters," who have repeatedly given me the gift of undoing aloneness

—Hanna Levenson

Contents

Series Preface   ix
Tony Rousmaniere and Alexandre Vaz

Acknowledgments   xiii

Part I   Overview and Instructions   1

CHAPTER 1. Introduction and Overview of Deliberate Practice and
Accelerated Experiential Dynamic Psychotherapy   3

CHAPTER 2. Instructions for the Accelerated Experiential Dynamic
Psychotherapy Deliberate Practice Exercises   19

**Part II   Deliberate Practice Exercises for Accelerated
Experiential Dynamic Psychotherapy Skills   23**

*Exercises for Beginner Accelerated Experiential Dynamic
Psychotherapy Skills*

EXERCISE 1. Moment-to-Moment Tracking   25

EXERCISE 2. Exploring and Staying With Physical Experience   37

EXERCISE 3. Undoing Aloneness   53

EXERCISE 4. Affirming   63

*Exercises for Intermediate Accelerated Experiential Dynamic
Psychotherapy Skills*

EXERCISE 5. Self-Involving Self-Disclosure   73

EXERCISE 6. Self-Revealing Self-Disclosure   85

EXERCISE 7. Metaprocessing   95

*Exercises for Advanced Accelerated Experiential Dynamic
Psychotherapy Skills*

EXERCISE 8. Working With Anxiety   107

EXERCISE 9. Affirmative Work With Defenses   119

EXERCISE 10. Initiating Portrayals   131

EXERCISE 11. Privileging Transformation Strivings   143

EXERCISE 12. Metatherapeutic Processing   157

Comprehensive Exercises

EXERCISE 13. Annotated Accelerated Experiential Dynamic Psychotherapy Practice
Session Transcript   183

EXERCISE 14. Mock Accelerated Experiential Dynamic Psychotherapy Sessions   191

Part III   Strategies for Enhancing the Deliberate Practice Exercises   199

CHAPTER 3. How to Get the Most Out of Deliberate Practice: Additional Guidance for
Trainers and Trainees   201

APPENDIX A. Difficulty Assessments and Adjustments   215

APPENDIX B. Deliberate Practice Diary Form   219

APPENDIX C. Sample Accelerated Experiential Dynamic Psychotherapy Syllabus With
Embedded Deliberate Practice Exercises   223

References   231

Index   241

About the Authors   245

Series Preface

Tony Rousmaniere and Alexandre Vaz

We are pleased to introduce the Essentials of Deliberate Practice series of training books. We are developing this series to address a specific need that we see in many psychology training programs. The issue can be illustrated by the training experiences of Mary, a hypothetical second-year graduate school trainee. Mary has learned a lot about mental health theory, research, and psychotherapy techniques. Mary is a dedicated student; she has read dozens of textbooks, written excellent papers about psychotherapy, and receives near-perfect scores on her course exams. However, when Mary sits with her clients at her practicum site, she often has trouble performing the therapy skills that she can write and talk about so clearly. Furthermore, Mary has noticed herself getting anxious when her clients express strong reactions, such as getting very emotional, hopeless, or skeptical about therapy. Sometimes this anxiety is strong enough to make Mary freeze at key moments, limiting her ability to help those clients.

During her weekly individual and group supervision, Mary's supervisor gives her advice informed by empirically supported therapies and common factor methods. The supervisor often supplements that advice by leading Mary through role plays, recommending additional reading, or providing examples from her own work with clients. Mary, a dedicated supervisee who shares tapes of her sessions with her supervisor, is open about her challenges, carefully writes down her supervisor's advice, and reads the suggested readings. However, when Mary sits back down with her clients, she often finds that her new knowledge seems to have flown out of her head, and she is unable to enact her supervisor's advice. Mary finds this problem to be particularly acute with the clients who are emotionally evocative.

Mary's supervisor, who has received formal training in supervision, uses supervisory best practices, including the use of video to review supervisees' work. She would rate Mary's overall competence level as consistent with expectations for a trainee at Mary's developmental level. But even though Mary's overall progress is positive, she experiences some recurring problems in her work. This is true even though the supervisor is confident that she and Mary have identified the changes that Mary should make in her work.

The problem with which Mary and her supervisor are wrestling—the disconnect between her knowledge about psychotherapy and her ability to reliably perform psychotherapy—is the focus of this book series. We started this series because most therapists experience this disconnect, to one degree or another, whether they are beginning trainees or highly experienced clinicians. In truth, we are all Mary.

To address this problem, we are focusing this series on the use of deliberate practice, a method of training specifically designed for improving reliable performance of complex skills in challenging work environments (Rousmaniere, 2016, 2019; Rousmaniere et al., 2017). Deliberate practice entails experiential, repeated training with a particular skill until it becomes automatic. In the context of psychotherapy, this involves two trainees role-playing as a client and a therapist, switching roles every so often, under the guidance of a supervisor. The trainee playing the therapist reacts to client statements, ranging in difficulty from beginner to intermediate to advanced, with improvised responses that reflect fundamental therapeutic skills.

To create these books, we approached leading trainers and researchers of major therapy models with these simple instructions: Identify 10 to 12 essential skills for your therapy model where trainees often experience a disconnect between cognitive knowledge and performance ability—in other words, skills that trainees could write a good paper about but often have challenges performing, especially with challenging clients. We then collaborated with the authors to create deliberate practice exercises specifically designed to improve reliable performance of these skills and overall responsive treatment (Hatcher, 2015; Stiles et al., 1998; Stiles & Horvath, 2017). Finally, we rigorously tested these exercises with trainees and trainers at multiple sites around the world and refined them based on extensive feedback.

Each book in this series focuses on a specific therapy model, but readers will notice that most exercises in these books touch on common factor variables and facilitative interpersonal skills that researchers have identified as having the most impact on client outcome, such as empathy, verbal fluency, emotional expression, persuasiveness, and problem focus (e.g., Anderson et al., 2009; Norcross et al., 2019). Thus, the exercises in every book should help with a broad range of clients. Despite the specific theoretical model(s) from which therapists work, most therapists place a strong emphasis on pantheoretical elements of the therapeutic relationship, many of which have robust empirical support as correlates or mechanisms of client improvement (e.g., Norcross et al., 2019). We also recognize that therapy models have established training programs with rich histories, so we present deliberate practice not as a replacement but as an adaptable, transtheoretical training method that can be integrated into these existing programs to improve skill retention and help ensure basic competency.

About This Book

This book in the series is on accelerated experiential dynamic psychotherapy (AEDP), an integrative model of psychotherapy that focuses on the positive experience of corrective emotional and relational interactions within sessions and session to session, not only to alleviate suffering (like many psychotherapy models) but also to enhance functioning and encourage "flourishing" (Fosha, 2000, 2017a; Fosha & Thoma, 2020). Its methods center on relational dynamics to undo aloneness, and draw on advances in attachment and emotion theory, affective neuroscience, and positive psychology.

A trainee may read about AEDP and be knowledgeable about the theory of AEDP, but this knowledge often does not translate to skillful implementation of AEDP practices. Practicing AEDP skills, with ongoing feedback, is needed to build and deepen a clinician's use of AEDP in clinical settings.

In this book, we adopt deliberate practice methods to support experiential—learn by doing—training opportunities. The described methods and prompts facilitate practicing a range of important AEDP skills. In addition, it supports fine-tuning the "how" of intervention delivery, including in a flexible manner across diverse clinical scenarios. Importantly, this book is not intended to replace AEDP training courses and their exposure to foundational AEDP theory and principles of practice. Rather, it is intended to augment training programs.

Thank you for including us in your journey toward psychotherapy expertise. Now let's get to practice!

Acknowledgments

We would like to acknowledge Rodney Goodyear for his significant contribution to starting and organizing this book series. We are grateful to Susan Reynolds, David Becker, Elizabeth Budd, Elizabeth Brace, and Emily Ekle at American Psychological Association (APA) Books for providing expert guidance and insightful editing that has significantly improved the quality and accessibility of this book. We would also like to acknowledge the International Deliberate Practice Society and its members for their many contributions and support for our work.

I (Natasha Prenn) would like to thank my mentors and friends: Diana Fosha, Ben Lipton, Ron Frederick, Judith Ruskay Rabinor, and Charles Rowan Beye. I also thank my true others: Jeanne Newhouse, Kate Halliday, Hilary Jacobs Hendel, and Jessica Slatus. I dedicate this book to Hanna Levenson and Alexandre Vaz: working with them made the writing of this book a profoundly transformational experience.

I (Hanna Levenson) acknowledge the gift of time from the Wright Institute to devote to this project. The administrative and editing help from Rajika Mehra was invaluable. I also thank my patients, students, colleagues, mentors, friends, and family for their support and contributions in so many diverse and unexpected ways over the years. A particular shout-out goes to Craig McAllister for his graciousness in understanding my nose being in my computer for more time than I would like to admit.

The exercises in this book series have undergone extensive testing at multiple training programs. For everyone who volunteered to "test run" this work and provided critically important feedback throughout the method refinement and writing process, we cannot thank you enough.

We would particularly like to acknowledge these colleagues for volunteering to test exercises: Elina Alexandrov, Gemma Armstrong, Jamie Bachman, Jessey Bernstein, Melanie Carter, Kevin Felix, Jessica Guillory, Dagmar Kaufmann, Sara Kranzler, Catherine McLaughlin, and Elley Newton. And much appreciation goes to the attendees of the workshop in Ithaca, New York, with Kate Halliday: Sally Ryan, Donna George, Snowy Lajoie, Jenn Heatley, Casey Benson, Jenny Grabelsky, Jacob White, Suki Hall, Laurie Buehler, J McKnight, Nadia Grigg, Thaddeus Bates, Hannah Rumpf, Dalya Tamir, Elley Newton, Catherine, Shane Alison Bliss, Jennifer Marshall, Lisa Strayer, and Laura Ward.

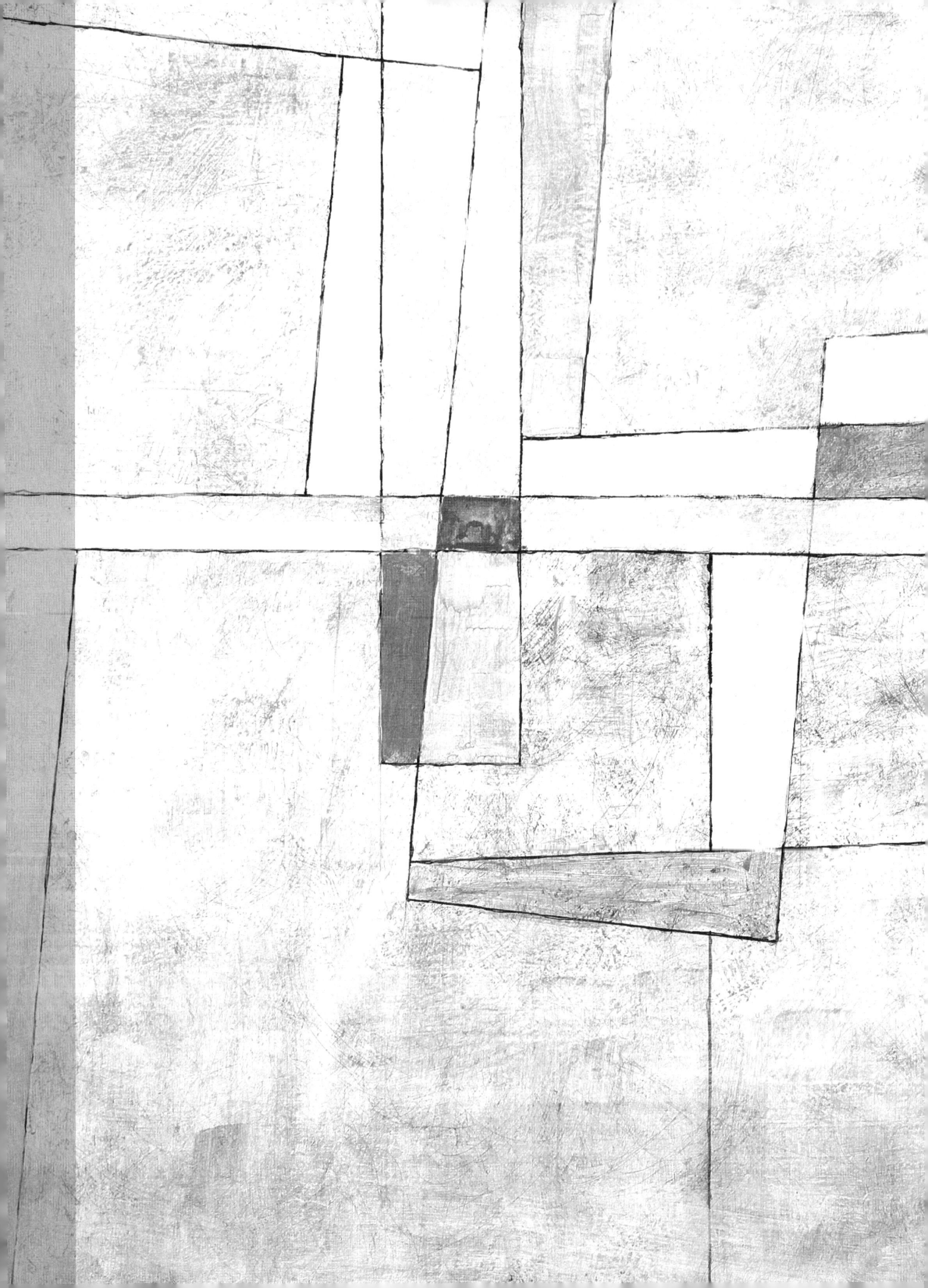

Overview and Instructions

In Part I, we provide an overview of deliberate practice, including how it can be integrated into clinical training programs for accelerated experiential dynamic psychotherapy (AEDP), and instructions for performing the deliberate practice exercises in Part II. **We encourage both trainers and trainees to read both Chapters 1 and 2 before performing the deliberate practice exercises for the first time.**

Chapter 1 provides a foundation for the rest of the book by introducing important concepts related to deliberate practice and its role in psychotherapy training more broadly and AEDP training more specifically. We also individually review the 12 skills from these exercises.

Chapter 2 lays out the basic, most essential instructions for performing the AEDP deliberate practice exercises in Part II. They are designed to be quick and simple and provide you with just enough information to get started without being overwhelmed by too much information. Chapter 3 in Part III provides more in-depth guidance, which we encourage you to read once you are comfortable with the basic instructions in Chapter 2.

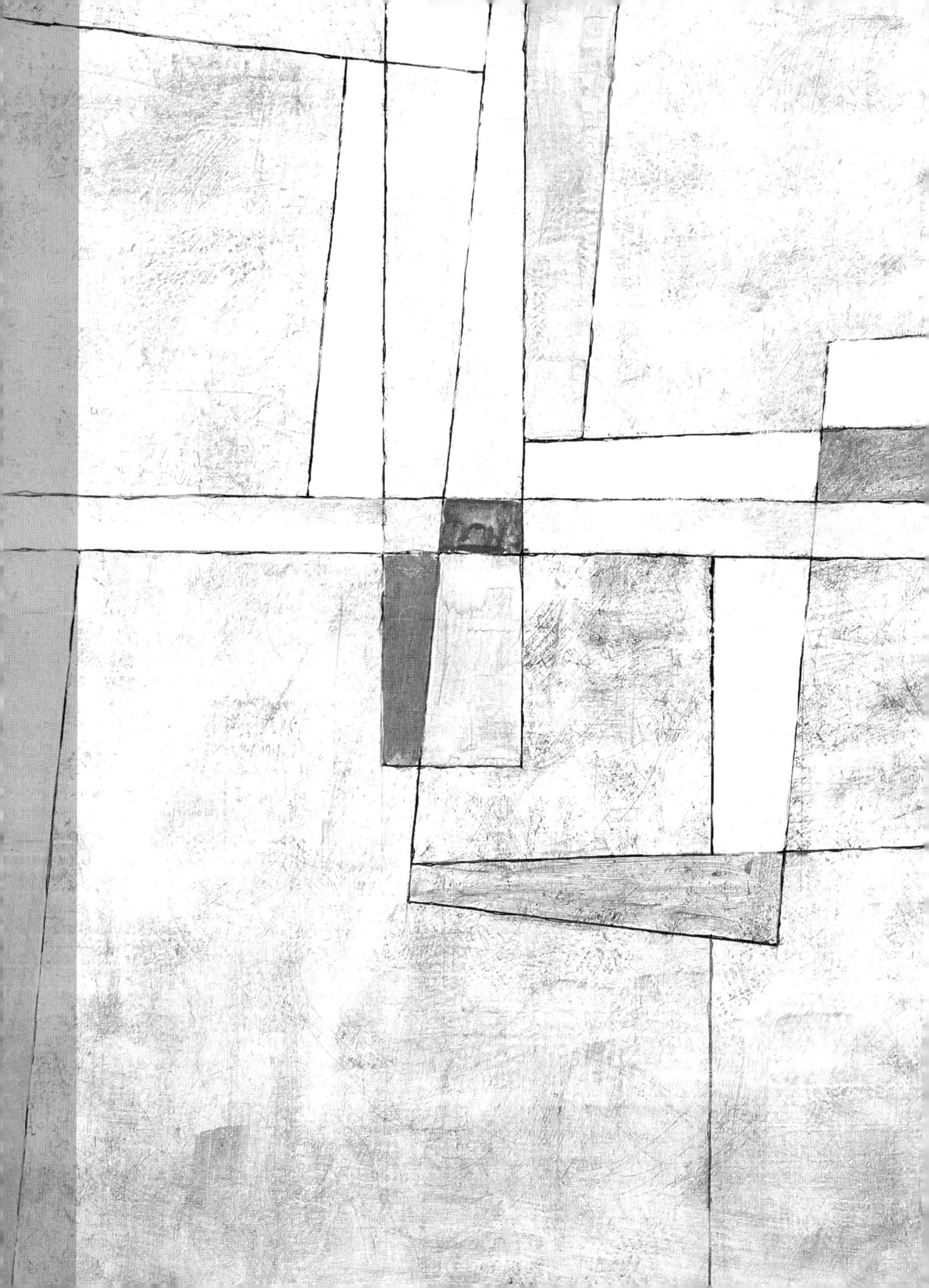

Introduction and Overview of Deliberate Practice and Accelerated Experiential Dynamic Psychotherapy

I (Natasha Prenn) am fortunate to have come to accelerated experiential dynamic psychotherapy (AEDP) early in my career change from a teacher of Latin and ancient Greek to psychotherapist. I did not have to "unlearn" other ways of working therapeutically. Yet as I started my psychotherapy training, I asked over and over again, "I understand the theory but what do I say and do in session with clients?" I was always struck by how few examples of words that psychotherapists actually said were included in otherwise useful books. Over the years, this led to my compiling lists of interventions and things to say when I was reading psychotherapy books. Within the AEDP community, I became known and teased for my notebook of interventions.

Fortunately for me, when I found AEDP, not only were there videotapes of sessions to watch and from which I could copy interventions, there were also transcripts in every AEDP article so that I could select interventions to practice and experiment with. Relying on my background as a language teacher, I started to put together the best and most effective interventions in a workshop I called "What Do I Say? How Do I Say It? And Then What Do I Do?—AEDP and Experiential Language." I discovered that there are some interventions that work reliably and can be used and reused to great effect.

On top of this, I also had my own experiences in psychoanalysis where my analyst made a brilliant interpretation almost every session, but I didn't get much better. My AEDP therapist said some version of "stay with it, and stay with me" every session, and that seemed to help me a lot!

By this time, I was a faculty member at the AEDP Institute in New York City. My compilation of the most productive interventions coincided with the development of the AEDP Essential Skills courses where we taught AEDP through the nuts and bolts of what a therapist actually says—one skill at a time. It was deliberate practice lite! More than one course participant described it as ballet steps that they practiced over and over again until they had it in their bones and could then improvise. So when Hanna invited me to join her in writing this book, I jumped at the chance to upgrade deliberate practice lite into a full-fledged, formal book of deliberate practice for learning AEDP skills.

https://doi.org/10.1037/0000439-001

Deliberate Practice in Accelerated Experiential Dynamic Psychotherapy, by N. C. N. Prenn, H. Levenson, A. Vaz, and T. Rousmaniere

And I (Hanna Levenson) was so excited that Natasha took me up on my invitation! She was *the* person I wanted to collaborate with on this project; the materials she created for AEDP were so helpful to me in learning the model. Even before I met Natasha 15 years ago, I knew we were kindred spirits with our zeal for preciseness, simplicity, and clarity in making the implicit explicit and in making the explicit teachable.

I came to AEDP after many years of working on a model of time-limited dynamic psychotherapy (TLDP; Levenson, 1995, 2017). In my approach to TLDP, I privileged experiential learning (especially corrective emotional experiences between the therapist and the patient) over insight, and focused on emotional processing, influenced by decades of doing emotionally focused couple therapy (Levenson et al., 2025). Was it any wonder that AEDP felt like the "whole package" to me: short term (accelerated), experiential, dynamic, and emotionally based with a focus on the therapeutic relationship?

From there I began taking AEDP trainings, helped Diana Fosha and her AEDP Institute Faculty construct the AEDP Fidelity Scale (Levenson et al., 2011), and conducted some research on the model (Faerstein et al., 2016). I then invited Natasha and Diana to write a book on AEDP supervision for a supervision series I was coediting for APA (Prenn & Fosha, 2017), and hosted and interviewed Diana about her supervision of a trainee—all of which was recorded for a professional video (Fosha & Levenson, 2016). I consider this book not only a culmination of those experiences but also a boon to my learning AEDP skills, illustrating the old saying that if you truly want to understand something, try to teach it to someone else.

Overview of the Deliberate Practice Exercises

The main focus of the book is a series of 14 exercises that have been tested and modified based on feedback from AEDP faculty, supervisors, and supervisees. The first 12 exercises each represent an essential AEDP skill. Exercises 13 and 14 are more comprehensive, consisting of an annotated AEDP transcript and improvised mock therapy sessions with six client profiles. Both these exercises are designed to facilitate the trainees' learning how to integrate the 12 essential skills into the flow of a real therapy session. In Exercise 14, we have tried to provide a diversity of client profiles in terms of age, race, religion, socio-economics, gender, and sexual orientation. We hope trainees[1] practicing these role plays will feel free to change the client profiles in ways that make them feel most comfortable. Table 1.1 presents the 12 skills that are covered in these exercises.

Throughout the exercises, trainees work in pairs under the guidance of a trainer and role-play as a client and a therapist, switching back and forth between the two roles. Each of the 12 skill-focused exercises consists of multiple client statements grouped by difficulty—beginner, intermediate, and advanced—that calls for a specific skill. For each skill, trainees are asked to read through and absorb the description of the skill, its criteria, and some examples of it. The trainee playing the client then reads the statements that present possible problems and emotional states, or client markers. The trainee playing the therapist then responds in a way that demonstrates the appropriate skill. Trainee therapists will have the option of practicing a response using the one supplied in the exercise or immediately improvising and supplying their own.

---

1. We use the generic words *trainer* and *trainee* throughout this book. In this way, *trainer* can refer to a teacher, professor, or instructor in the classroom who might be using the text, whereas in a different context, it can refer to a supervisor in a supervision session. Similarly, *trainee* can refer to a student in a classroom learning environment or a supervisee in a supervision session.

TABLE 1.1. The 12 Accelerated Experiential Dynamic Psychotherapy Skills Presented in the Deliberate Practice Exercises

Beginner Skills	Intermediate Skills	Advanced Skills
1. Moment-to-moment tracking 2. Exploring and staying with physical experience 3. Undoing aloneness 4. Affirming	5. Self-involving self-disclosure 6. Self-revealing self-disclosure 7. Metaprocessing	8. Working with anxiety 9. Affirmative work with defenses 10. Initiating portrayals 11. Privileging transformance strivings 12. Metatherapeutic processing

After each client statement and therapist response couplet is practiced several times, the trainees will stop to receive feedback from the trainer. Guided by the trainer, the trainees are instructed to try statement–response couplets several times, working their way down the list. In consultation with the trainer, trainees will go through the exercises, starting with the least challenging and moving through to more advanced levels. The triad (trainer–client–therapist) will have the opportunity to discuss whether exercises present too much or too little challenge and adjust up or down depending on the assessment.

Trainees, in consultation with trainers, can decide which skills they wish to work on and for how long. On the basis of our testing experience, we have found practice sessions last about 1 hour to receive maximum benefit. After this, trainees become saturated and need a break.

Ideally, AEDP learners will both gain confidence and achieve competence through practicing these exercises. Competence is defined here as the ability to perform an AEDP skill in a manner that is flexible and responsive to the client. Skills have been chosen that are considered essential to AEDP and that practitioners often find challenging to implement.

The skills identified in this book are not comprehensive in the sense of representing all one needs to learn to become a competent AEDP clinician. Some will present particular challenges for trainees. A short history of AEDP and a brief description of the deliberate practice methodology is provided to explain how we have arrived at the union between them.

The Goals of This Book

The primary goal of this book is to help trainees achieve competence in core AEDP skills. Therefore, the expression of that skill or competency may look somewhat different across clients or even within session with the same client.

The AEDP deliberate practice exercises are designed to achieve the following:

1. Help AEDP therapists develop the ability to apply the skills in a range of clinical situations.

2. Move the skills into procedural memory (Squire, 2004) so that AEDP therapists can access them reliably and automatically.

3. Provide AEDP therapists in training with an opportunity to exercise the particular skill using a style and language that is congruent with who they are.

4. Provide the opportunity to use the AEDP skills in response to varying client statements and affect. This is designed to build confidence to adopt skills in a broad range of circumstances within different client contexts.

5. Provide AEDP therapists in training with many opportunities to stumble and then correct their response based on feedback. This helps build confidence and persistence.

Finally, this book aims to help trainees discover their own personal learning style so that they can continue their professional development long after their formal training is concluded.

Who Can Benefit From This Book?

This book is designed to be used in multiple contexts, including in graduate-level courses, supervision, postgraduate training, and continuing education programs. It can also be used as a self-study book. (See some helpful hints about this in Chapter 3, "How to Get the Most Out of Deliberate Practice: Additional Guidance for Trainers and Trainees.") It assumes the following:

1. The trainer is knowledgeable about and competent in AEDP.

2. The trainer is able to provide good demonstrations of how to use AEDP skills across a range of therapeutic situations, via role play and/or video recording of excerpts of psychotherapy sessions.

3. The trainer is able to provide feedback to students regarding how to craft or improve their application of AEDP skills.

4. Trainees will have accompanying reading, such as books and articles, that explain the theory, research, and rationale of AEDP and each particular skill. Recommended reading for each skill is provided in the sample syllabus (Appendix C).

The exercises covered in this book were piloted in various training sites. This book is intended to be used by trainers and trainees from different cultural backgrounds worldwide. For guidance on how to improve one's skills in dealing with multicultural issues through deliberate practice, see *Deliberate Practice in Multicultural Therapy* (Harris et al., 2024).

This book is designed for those who are training at all career stages, from beginning trainees, including those who have never worked with real clients, to seasoned therapists. All exercises feature guidance for assessing and adjusting the difficulty to precisely target the needs of each individual learner. The term *trainee* in this book is used broadly, referring to anyone in the field of professional mental health who is endeavoring to acquire AEDP skills.

Deliberate Practice in Psychotherapy Training

How does one become an expert in their professional field? What is trainable and what is simply beyond our reach, due to innate or uncontrollable factors? Questions such as these touch on our fascination with expert performers and their development. What accounts for consistently superior professional results? Evidence suggests that the amount of time spent on a particular type of training is a key factor in developing expertise in virtually all domains (Ericsson & Pool, 2016). "Deliberate practice" is an evidence-based method that can improve performance in an effective and reliable manner.

The concept of deliberate practice has its origins in a classic study by K. Anders Ericsson and colleagues (1993). They found that the amount of time practicing a skill and the quality of the time spent doing so were key factors predicting mastery and acquisition. They identified five key activities in learning and mastering skills: (a) observing one's own work, (b) getting expert feedback, (c) setting small incremental learning goals just beyond the performer's ability, (d) engaging in repetitive behavioral rehearsal of specific skills, and (e) continuously assessing performance. Ericsson and his colleagues termed this process deliberate practice, a cyclical process that is illustrated in Figure 1.1.

Research has shown that lengthy engagement in deliberate practice is associated with expert performance across a variety of professional fields, such as medicine, sports, music, chess, computer programming, and mathematics (Ericsson et al., 2018). People may associate deliberate practice with the widely known "10,000-hour rule" popularized by Malcolm Gladwell in his 2008 book *Outliers*, although the actual number of hours required for expertise varies by field and by individual (Ericsson & Pool, 2016). This, however, perpetuated two misunderstandings. First, that this is the number of deliberate practice hours that everyone needs to attain expertise, no matter the domain. In fact, there can be considerable variability in how many hours are required.

The second misunderstanding is that engagement in 10,000 hours of work performance will lead one to become an expert in that domain. This misunderstanding holds considerable significance for the field of psychotherapy, where hours of work experience with clients has traditionally been used as a measure of proficiency (Rousmaniere, 2016). Research suggests that the amount of experience alone does not predict therapist effectiveness (Goldberg, Rousmaniere, et al., 2016). It may be that the quality of deliberate practice is a key factor.

Psychotherapy scholars, recognizing the value of deliberate practice in other fields, have called for deliberate practice to be incorporated into training for mental health

FIGURE 1.1. Cycle of Deliberate Practice

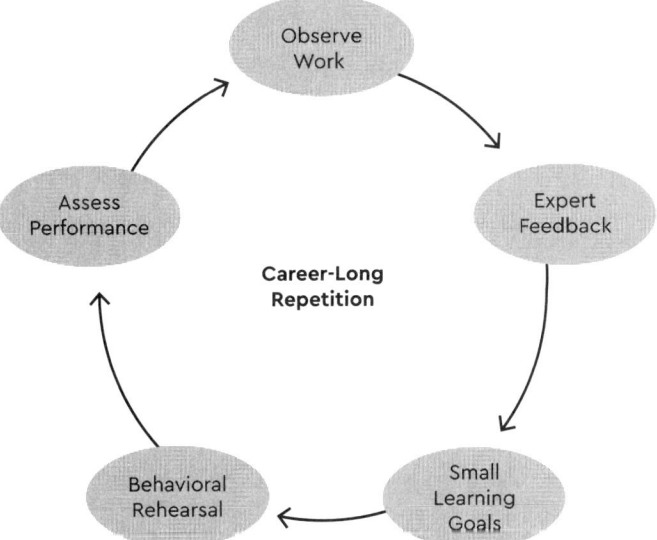

Note. From *Deliberate Practice in Emotion-Focused Therapy* (p. 7), by R. N. Goldman, A. Vaz, and T. Rousmaniere, 2021, American Psychological Association (https://doi.org/10.1037/0000227-000). Copyright 2021 by the American Psychological Association.

professionals (e.g., Bailey & Ogles, 2019; Hill et al., 2020; Rousmaniere et al., 2017; Taylor & Neimeyer, 2017; Tracey et al., 2015). There are, however, good reasons to question analogies made between psychotherapy and other professional fields such as sports or music because by comparison, psychotherapy is so complex and free-form. Sports have clearly defined goals, and classical music follows a written score. In contrast, the goals of psychotherapy shift with the unique presentation of each client at each session. Therapists do not have the luxury of following a score.

Instead, good psychotherapy is more like improvisation (Noa Kageyama, cited in Rousmaniere, 2016). In jazz improvisations, a complex mixture of group collaboration, creativity, and interaction are coconstructed among band members. Like psycho-therapy, no two jazz improvisations are identical. However, improvisations are not a random collection of notes. They are grounded in a comprehensive theoretical under-standing and technical proficiency that is only developed through continuous delib-erate practice. For example, prominent jazz instructor Jerry Coker (1990) listed 18 skill areas that students must master, each of which has multiple discrete skills including tone quality, intervals, chord arpeggios, scales, patterns, and licks. In this sense, more creative and artful improvisations are actually a reflection of a previous commitment to repetitive skill practice and acquisition. Legendary jazz musician Miles Davis summed it up: "You have to play a long time to be able to play like yourself" (Cook, 2005, p. 112).

The main idea that we would like to stress here is that we want deliberate practice to help AEDP therapists become themselves. The idea is to learn the skills so that you have them on hand when you want them. Practice the skills to make them your own. Incorporate those aspects that feel right for you. Ongoing and effortful deliberate prac-tice should not be an impediment to flexibility and creativity. Ideally, it should enhance it. We recognize and celebrate that psychotherapy is an ever-shifting encounter and by no means want it to become or feel formulaic. Strong AEDP therapists mix an eloquent integration of previously acquired skills with properly attuned flexibility. The core AEDP responses provided are meant as templates or possibilities, rather than "answers." Please interpret and apply them as you see fit, in a way that makes sense to you. We encourage flexible and improvisational play!

Simulation-Based Mastery Learning

Deliberate practice uses simulation-based mastery learning (Ericsson, 2004; McGaghie et al., 2014). That is, the stimulus material for training consists of "contrived social situa-tions that mimic problems, events, or conditions that arise in professional encounters" (McGaghie et al., 2014, p. 375). A key component of this approach is that the stimuli being used in training are sufficiently similar to the real-world experiences so that they mimic that they provoke similar reactions. This facilitates *state-dependent learning* in which professionals acquire skills in the same psychological environment where they will have to perform the skills (Fisher & Craik, 1977). For example, pilots train with flight simulators that present mechanical failures and dangerous weather conditions, and surgeons prac-tice with surgical simulators that present medical complications. Training in simulations with challenging stimuli increases professionals' capacity to perform effectively under stress. For the psychotherapy training exercises in this book, the "simulators" are typical client statements that might actually be presented in the course of therapy sessions and call on the use of the particular skill.

Declarative Versus Procedural Knowledge

Declarative knowledge is what a person can understand, write, or speak about. It often refers to factual information that can be consciously recalled through memory and is often acquired relatively quickly. In contrast, procedural learning is implicit in memory requiring *repetition of an activity*, which then is evidenced in *improved task performance* (Koziol & Budding, 2012). Procedural knowledge is what a person can perform, especially under stress (Squire, 2004). There can be a wide difference between their declarative and procedural knowledge. For example, an "armchair quarterback" is a person who understands and talks about athletics well but would have trouble performing it at a professional ability. Likewise, most dance, music, or theater critics have a very high ability to write about their subjects but would be flummoxed if asked to perform them.

The sweet spot for deliberate practice is the gap between declarative and procedural knowledge. In other words, effortful practice should target those skills that the trainee could write a good paper about but would have trouble actually performing with a real client. We start with declarative knowledge, learning skills theoretically and observing others perform them. Once learned, with the help of deliberate practice, we work toward the development of procedural learning, with the aim of therapists having "automatic" access to each of the skills that they can pull on when necessary.

Let us turn to a little theoretical background on AEDP to help contextualize the skills of the book and how they fit into the greater training model.

Overview of Accelerated Experiential Dynamic Psychotherapy

Healing oriented and attachment based, AEDP is a comprehensive integrative and transformative model of psychotherapy. Its experiential approach incorporates attachment research, emotion theory, experiential ways of working, transformational studies, developmental models, trauma approaches, body-focused treatments, and affective neuroscience. AEDP understands psychopathology as being the result of "unwilled and unwanted aloneness" in the face of emotionally overwhelming experience (Fosha, 2009, p. 182; Tunnel & Osiason, 2021, p. 89). To transform psychopathology and restore access to adaptive emotions, the AEDP therapist seeks relentlessly to undo the client's aloneness with explicitly relational, affirming, and self-disclosing interventions. With the visceral experience of knowing that there is a supportive, emotionally engaged other with whom to share both suffering and joys, the client can relinquish their reliance on defenses and begin to risk genuine emotional and relational experiencing, emotional processing, and healing.

AEDP has its lineage in psychodynamic psychotherapy and the short-term dynamic/experiential psychotherapies. However, in AEDP the attachment relationship is center stage. From the very first moments of the very first session, the AEDP therapist works to let the client know they are a team using an explicitly empathic, emotionally engaged, "we're in this together" stance.

AEDP has a very different lens and focus than most approaches to psychotherapy. We are looking for and have an understanding of what goes right and how to make things go right. In AEDP, we are always striving to help the client have a new experience and have that experience be a good one (Fosha, 2002). We often read that safety and attachment—a secure base—need to be in place before further work can be done. AEDP practitioners argue that corrective emotional and relational experiences in therapy create earned secure attachment (Prenn, 2009; Wallin, 2007), changing one's attachment status over time. In other words, secure attachment doesn't precede the work; it comes out of the process of the work.

We seek to establish a secure attachment relationship from the very beginning of each session by leading with risk taking—for example, our self-disclosures and vulnerability (Fosha, 2006; Lipton & Fosha, 2011; Prenn, 2009). This encourages clients to take more risks, and in this way the work becomes deeper. As therapist and client are able to traverse increasingly challenging moments together, the relationship becomes more solid, allowing therapist and client to take even more risks, and in this way the "thickness" of the relationship increases (Tronick, 1998).

There are two fundamental and overlapping maps that underpin all we are doing in AEDP and guide its process: the triangle of experience and the four-state model. The triangle of experience is a triangle standing on its point. It is most easily represented by raising your arms wide in a V-shape and imagining a line between your hands forming a triangle. In your right hand is the defense angle of the triangle, and in your left hand is the anxiety angle. Your heart in your chest is the bottom of the triangle where core feelings and core relational experiences live (see Figure 1.2). In AEDP, we help clients move from defense and anxiety down into their core feelings. With this image in mind, AEDP therapists are guided in all their interventions: feeling core feelings in the context of a secure attachment with another person is transformational.

With regard to the four-state model, the therapist helps the client gently move out of a place of anxiety and defense (what we call State 1) down into core feeling and core relational experiences (State 2). Once the therapist and client have dropped down into State 2 together, they process what it feels like (metatherapeutic processing, State 3). From this place of reflecting on what it feels like to experience deep and core emotions, we can notice that it feels good to do it together—even if at times painful— arriving at core state (State 4), a place of ease and clarity, typified by "This is me and I am okay." During this stage, the client often experiences a sense of a wise, authentic self-connection to the universe and everything in it. With this in mind, as you learn the 12 skills, think about where each one is positioned from the perspective of the triangle of experience and the four-state model.

FIGURE 1.2. Triangle of Experience

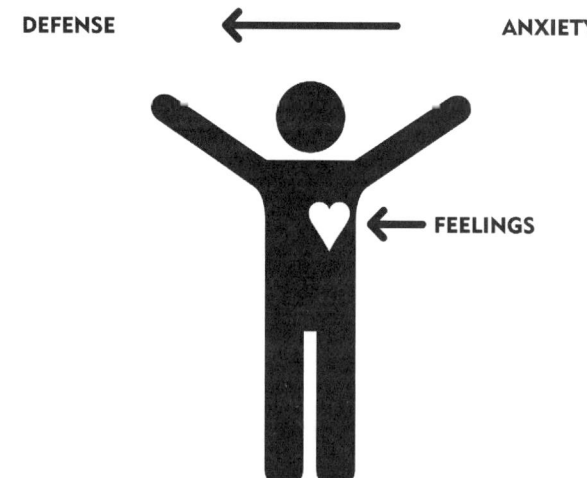

Note. The triangle of experience here is depicted by a person with arms raised and holding defenses in their right hand and anxieties in their left. These join together at the heart, the tip of the inverted triangle, which represents a person's core feelings and core relational experiences. Adapted from *Supervision Essentials for Accelerated Experiential Dynamic Psychotherapy* (p. 34), by N. C. N. Prenn and D. Fosha, 2017, American Psychological Association (https://doi.org/10.1037/0000016–000). Copyright 2016 by Victor Koen. Adapted with permission.

Accelerated Experiential Dynamic Psychotherapy Research

Although empirical investigations of AEDP's processes and outcomes "have only just begun" (Iwakabe et al., 2020, p. 550), there are already some impressive clinical research findings. Systematic case studies have been conducted (e.g., Blimling, 2019a; Gonzalez, 2018b; Markin et al., 2018) with commentaries (e.g., Fosha, 2018; Harrison, 2019; Iwakabe, 2018; Skean, 2018) and replies to the commentaries (e.g., Blimling, 2019b; Gonzalez, 2018a), illustrating AEDP's ability to facilitate emotional change processes as applied to specific clinical cases. In addition to case studies, task analyses of AEDP interventions have been qualitatively described (Iwakabe & Conceicao, 2016; Lee, 2015), outlining the essential ingredients and processes of AEDP interventions (e.g., metaprocesses and metatherapeutic processing).

Initial support of the effectiveness of AEDP comes from an outcome study of 62 adults receiving a 16-session version of AEDP treatment that occurred in naturalistic, private practice, outpatient settings in the United States, Canada, Israel, Japan, and Sweden (Iwakabe et al., 2020). According to the authors of this study,

> Therapists were instructed to use the AEDP framework actively to optimize the therapeutic relationship and facilitate patients' experiential processing of emotional, relational, and transformational experiences (Fosha, 2013; Prenn & Fosha, 2016). Therapist intervention strategies included: (a) focusing on and working with glimmers of transformance from the get-go; (b) strategies to restructure or bypass patient defenses; (c) dyadic affect regulation and other relational strategies aimed at building relational capacities; (d) experiential-affective strategies to process patients' painful emotions; and (e) metatherapeutic processing strategies to deepen and expand the emerging positive affective experiences associated with transformational experiences. (p. 435)

After treatment, most of the patients experienced significantly less distress, and significant improvement in their positive psychological functioning, achieving large effect sizes ($d > .80$), indicating clinically reliable change. These posttreatment outcome results are consistent with AEDP's aim of alleviating suffering while promoting flourishing.

Using the same sample, Iwakabe and colleagues (2022) examined AEDP's long-term effectiveness (Iwakabe et al., 2022). For both 6-month ($N = 40$) and 12-month ($N = 52$) follow-ups, patients maintained their gains. Large effect sizes were obtained ($d = 0.74$–1.60) for both lessening distress (e.g., depression, negative automatic thoughts, experiential avoidance) and increasing positive mental health (e.g., well-being, self-compassion). Furthermore, the patients reporting the most severe problems had even larger effect sizes. Thus, for both immediate and long-term outcome, AEDP as practiced in "real-world" treatment settings achieved results similar to those found for emotion-focused therapy, short-term dynamic psychotherapy, and cognitive behavioral therapy. "This is particularly notable in that AEDP focuses on in-session change rather than the direct teaching of coping skills and between-session skills practice" (Iwakabe et al., 2022, p. 442). The authors did note that the absence of a control group meant that certain factors (e.g., regression toward the mean) were not controlled.

In looking at the relationship between the working therapeutic alliance and positive emotions in a different sample, Notsu and colleagues (2023) found that higher positive emotions at the end of a session were predictive of better working alliances at the end of the next session. The authors concluded that "patients' experience of positive emotions has a significant role in strengthening the working alliance over the course of therapy" (p. 337).

Levenson, Fosha, and faculty members of the AEDP Institute (2011) constructed a scale to measure therapists' adherence to the AEDP stance and using AEDP interventions. The AEDP Fidelity Scale (AEDP-FS) was designed to capture "what makes AEDP, AEDP." Research with the AEDP-FS (Faerstein et al., 2016) shows good predictive and construct validity: The scale is measuring AEDP-specific and not general clinical skills; a 5-day AEDP training significantly increases participants' knowledge and competency; the ability to identify and evaluate one's feelings is significantly related to proficiency in AEDP; and a factor analysis of the scale reveals most of the items relate to AEDP's transformational processes.

Accelerated Experiential Dynamic Psychotherapy Skills in Deliberate Practice

All 12 of the skills in this book come down to two central principles in AEDP: that we can do with a trusted other what we cannot do alone and that symptoms and suffering come from clients' best attempts to handle overwhelming emotion and experience alone. The phrase "stay with it and stay with me" best sums up AEDP therapists' interventions (Pando-Mars & Fosha, 2025).

Imagine driving alone on a winding country road. You aren't sure you are on the right road and are feeling lost. Now imagine that a trusted friend is in the passenger seat saying, "We'll find our way. What an adventure we are on together!" Very different experiences. This is the essential core of AEDP. When we as therapists invite our clients to stay with it (their internal physical experience) and to stay with us (their therapists), we catapult ourselves into whatever the "it" is that has created the need for anxiety and defense around feelings in the dynamics of the relationship.

In the "undoing of aloneness," we try to give the client a new experience. For example, a client feels overwhelmed by feelings in their body and has learned to handle these feelings alone. As a child, no one helped them or soothed them when they felt sad, so now they might smile and say they're fine or make jokes and avoid their sadness. The cost of this protective strategy over time is that they do not get the benefits that come from knowing that they can feel sad, share their tears and sad feelings with another, and receive comfort. In AEDP, we try to give the client a new experience of staying with whatever feeling was feared and avoided ("stay with it"), helping them learn that they are capable of facing it now because they are not alone. The therapist ("stay with me") is not one of those people who can't handle their sadness. The therapist explicitly wants to be alongside the client when they have big feelings. AEDP says, "We can do together now what you could not do alone then." So as we review each of these 12 skills that you will learn or become more proficient in, keep in mind that each of them exemplifies these two central AEDP principles: staying with it and staying with me.

The Accelerated Experiential Dynamic Psychotherapy Skills Presented in Exercises 1 Through 12

Beginner Skills

Skill 1: Moment-to-Moment Tracking

Moment-to-moment tracking is a skill from which everything else in AEDP stems. It is the zoom-in, tight focus into the here-and-now of the client with the therapist. The therapist gently tracks the client's nonverbal movements and paraverbals, knowing that in this "talk therapy," the body is communicating just as much, if not more, than the words. It is through moment-to-moment tracking that we notice entry points, sense and name the reactions of our clients, and help what has been called the "unthought known" (Bollas, 1987) become center stage in our therapeutic work. This skill will help you and the client figure out what the "it" of "stay with it is."

Skill 2: Exploring and Staying With Physical Experience

In this exercise, we are focusing on two skills that get used in combination so frequently that we are presenting them together in this skill. The first skill component is exploring the client's physical experience, and the second is inviting the client to stay with that experience. Focusing the client on how they physically experience emotions, and helping them stay with that experience, results in more awareness of whatever is coming up inside. Because we are asking the client two questions, the exercise is in a dialogue format like a typical therapist–client exchange.

Skill 3: Undoing Aloneness

The importance of this skill was emphasized earlier. Undoing aloneness is a critical skill in AEDP. As therapists, we make it clear and explicit that we are with the client. We can do this in three ways: (a) with our body language and paraverbals, (b) by using "we" language and actually saying that we are with the client, and (c) by explicitly inquiring about the client's sense of our presence.

Skill 4: Affirming

The AEDP therapist is supportive, validating, and emotionally engaged from the first moments of the first session and throughout the therapy. Affirming is an intervention that promotes safety and trust by acknowledging and validating the client's experiences, strengths, and emotions. What you will learn in doing this skill is to be specific in what you are affirming and to match your vocal tone and nonverbal behavior to your affirming words. Often part of that specificity includes the therapist's self-disclosing how they are affected by what the client is saying, which leads us to the next skill.

Intermediate Skills

Skill 5: Self-Involving Self-Disclosure

There are two main kinds of self-disclosure. The first, self-involving self-disclosure, happens when the therapist describes their own affect and process, usually in response to something verbal or nonverbal the client expresses, as it unfolds in the session and from session to session. Here again, the therapist makes things explicit and specific. Interventions that demonstrate this skill often use the following format: "When I, the therapist, [see, feel, or sense] you do X, then I feel Y."

Skill 6: Self-Revealing Self-Disclosure

For this exercise, we use some of the same client statements as in the previous exercise, but for practicing a different skill. Self-revealing self-disclosures are when the therapist shares something personal about their own experience that relates to the essence of what the client is saying. It is a way of saying, "I have walked in your shoes." In AEDP, whenever possible we pair such self-disclosure with metaprocessing (Skill 7)—asking the client about how hearing this personal information affects them. Because these self-revealing self-disclosures are personal, they can be quite impactful on the therapeutic process. In the therapy hour, AEDP therapists use these interventions sparingly. Here, however, in the spirit of deliberate practice, you will get to repeatedly practice this skill.

Skill 7: Metaprocessing

Metaprocessing is used to focus on a very specific moment that is happening between therapist and patient, and inquire about it, without trying to figure it out or having preconceived ideas about what it might mean. This is a skill we use frequently in AEDP. Think of it as an "add-on" to almost any of the other skills to check out how the client is experiencing what is happening in the therapy. The standard format for a metaprocessing question is: "So what is this like for you right now that I noticed X or said Y or did Z]?" This is often the next intervention to almost everything we do in AEDP because what is critical is how the client experiences what is going on in the therapy for each specific intervention; metaprocessing helps keep the therapist and client in sync and on track, together.

Advanced Skills

Skill 8: Working With Anxiety

Anxiety tells us something important is coming up. Using this skill, we first focus on (re)educating clients that, from the perspective of emotion theory, anxiety can be an informative place for understanding when and why we are avoiding certain activities, thoughts, and feelings. Second, we ask permission of the client to explore their experience of anxiety. The goal of this skill is to help clients experience anxiety as a healthy signal from their bodies and not something to be feared, suppressed, or medicated away at its first signs.

Skill 9: Affirmative Work With Defenses

Many clients present in therapy relying on defensive strategies that helped them at one phase of their lives but now are not working, or are overworking, which causes symptoms and problems. In affirmatively working with defenses, you will practice naming what the client does instead of feeling primary affect, and then explicitly appreciating, even celebrating, the client's defense against feeling that affect. The third step is inviting the client to explore the defense or to bypass the defense, thereby opening up other possibilities. This is perhaps one of the most complex skills in the book.

Skill 10: Initiating Portrayals

A portrayal is a role-play technique that sets up a monologue or interaction either interpersonally through addressing an imagined person (real or fictitious), or with a part of the self. Portrayals are used to rework or complete "unfinished business" with another or with the self or work an unprocessed emotion such as anger or grief to completion. Practicing this skill will help you learn how to set up the conditions for this imagined dialogue. It is one of the ways we work with primary emotion in AEDP.

Skill 11: Privileging Transformance Strivings

Transformance is an individual's innate drive to be transformed—to right one's self, to grow, to be authentic and be known, connected, and recognized by the other. In privileging transformance strivings, AEDP therapists try to set up conditions for transformance to come to the fore. This skill involves looking out for glimmers of something positive in the client, and then using one of the 10 previous AEDP skills outlined in this book to promote that healthier behavior. This skill allows you to incorporate other skills you have already practiced and use them to promote growth.

Skill 12: Metatherapeutic Processing

This skill focuses on processing the experience of what is therapeutic about therapy. The goal is to help clients reflect on and take in the positive experience of change for the better. The format here is a therapist–client dialogue in which the therapist asks the client an open-ended question about a positive shift that they have mentioned. After the client has replied with their scripted statement, the therapist continues to ask open-ended questions focusing on deepening the client's experience of positive change.

A Note About Vocal Tone, Facial Expression, and Body Posture

In AEDP, we not only pay attention to the words we say to clients; we also pay exquisite attention to how we use our voice (e.g., tone, pitch, pacing, rhythm), our facial expressions (e.g., animated, still), and nonverbal behavior (e.g., body position, gestures, movement). With regard to the use of our voice in AEDP, we need a variety of tones and different speeds. We go slow and drop our voices into low, soothing tones to invite clients to move out of their thinking heads (usually in State 1—anxiety and defense) and into their bodies, hearts and feelings (Schore, 2001, 2009). Slowing down is a "foundational skill" in experiential work (Prenn & Fosha, 2017, p. 53). When clients slow down, they have a better chance to connect with their inner experience. Greenberg et al. (1993, p. 346) have underscored how critical a therapist's "experiential presence," conveyed through vocal tone and paraverbal expression, is for fostering positive outcomes—not just as a reflection of empathy but also as an expression of the therapist's own experience (Geller, 2020; Lipton, 2020; Prenn & Halliday, 2020). Another tone of voice the AEDP therapist needs is that which indicates delight and celebratory enthusiasm for the client's progress, imbuing words with the dynamic energy behind the exclamation points: "You did it! We did it together!" These ways to use the voice and body take some getting used to and refinement if you are only accustomed to the calm, evenly paced "therapist voice" accompanied by a nonexpressive face and still body.

All of this said, attunement is the key in all we do. If a new client is drawn into themselves in a hunched over position with little movement, we might quiet our own bodies to be in sync with them. If a client is energetic and smiling, we might engage likewise. This is not to say that we merely mirror a client; that is not attunement. Ideally, we will get to sense if a client's excitement is genuine or is covering a sadness they are afraid to feel or show us (or both). If the latter, we might try validating small shifts toward genuine feelings. In any case, our goal is to help clients feel successful in therapy; what we don't want to do is communicate that our clients are doing it wrong if they can't slow down or don't know what to make of the sensations and feelings in their bodies. While I (N. P.) was learning AEDP, I found Russell's (2007) suggestion helpful: "Feel yourself at the bottom of the triangle of experience (State 2 Core Feelings) and invite your client to join you there." If you remember the physical representation of the triangle described earlier, it is where your heart is.

In addition, AEDP learners will find it invaluable to watch recorded examples of expert AEDP therapists in session, so that they can observe these paraverbal and nonverbal interventions in action. It is important to watch as many AEDP therapists as possible so you can get a sense of how each AEDP therapist has their own unique manner for expressing their therapeutic presence. See the AEDP website for a list of such videos (https://aedpinstitute.org/apa-video-publications/).

The Role of Deliberate Practice in Accelerated Experiential Dynamic Psychotherapy Training

Since 1997 and even before, Diana Fosha has been unpacking and making explicit how to practice AEDP. Her 5-day Immersion Course (launched in 2003) immerses trainees in the experience of AEDP right from the very first moments of the very first meeting—rather like an actual AEDP therapy session. Almost immediately, small experiential groups start using AEDP interventions in role-play practice exercises.

In 2008, a few AEDP faculty members had a now famous conversation around my (N. P.'s) kitchen table and came up with the first AEDP Essential Skills Course, which launched 2 years later. Eventually this course evolved and expanded into Essential Skills Courses and Advanced Skills Modules. All these trainings focus heavily on the actual language of AEDP interventions and on lots of practice saying and doing and experiencing AEDP, albeit not in the precise form of this current book. In addition, individual and group AEDP supervision has used various intervention practice sheets and measures like the AEDP Fidelity Scale to keep the supervision on task. In essence, what we have found is that deliberate practice as a theory and a procedure integrates into the existing AEDP training program hand-in-glove. In the AEDP training, we have already been focusing on experiential practice in what might be called "deliberate practice lite." Now it is exciting to imagine how a full-scale application of deliberate practice methods and procedures will make the AEDP trainings even more beneficial.

Overview of the Book's Structure

This book is organized into three parts. Part I contains this chapter and Chapter 2, which provides basic instructions on how to perform these exercises. We found through testing that providing too many instructions upfront overwhelmed trainers and trainees, and as a result, they skipped past them. Therefore, we kept these instructions as brief and simple as possible to focus on only the most essential information that trainers and trainees will need to get started with the exercises. Further guidelines for getting the most about deliberate practice are provided in Chapter 3, and additional instructions for monitoring and adjusting the difficulty of the exercises are provided in Appendix A. **Do not skip the instructions in Chapter 2, and be sure to read the additional guidelines and instructions in Chapter 3 and Appendix A once you are comfortable with the basic instructions.**

Part II contains the 12 skill-focused exercises, which are ordered based on their difficulty: beginner, intermediate, and advanced (see Table 1.1). They each contain a brief overview of the exercise, example client–therapist interactions to help guide trainees, step-by-step instructions for conducting that exercise, and a list of criteria for mastering the relevant skill. The client statements and sample therapist responses are then presented, also organized by difficulty (beginner, intermediate, and advanced). The statements and responses are presented separately so that the trainee playing the therapist has more freedom to improvise responses without being influenced by the sample responses, which should only be turned to if the trainee has difficulty improvising their own responses. The last two exercises in Part II provide opportunities to practice the 12 skills within simulated psychotherapy sessions. Exercise 13 provides a sample psychotherapy session transcript in which the AEDP skills are used and clearly labeled, thereby demonstrating how they might flow together in an actual therapy session. AEDP trainees are invited to run through the sample transcript with one person playing the therapist and the other playing the client to get a feel for how a session might unfold. Exercise 14 provides suggestions for undertaking mock sessions, as well as client profiles ordered by difficulty (beginner, intermediate, and advanced) that trainees can use for improvised role plays.

Part III contains Chapter 3, which provides additional guidance for trainers and trainees. While Chapter 2 is more procedural, Chapter 3 covers big-picture issues. It highlights six key points for getting the most out of deliberate practice and describes the importance of appropriate responsiveness, attending to trainee well-being and respecting their privacy, and trainer self-evaluation, among other topics.

Three appendixes conclude this book. Appendix A provides instructions for monitoring and adjusting the difficulty of each exercise as needed. It provides a Deliberate Practice Reaction Form for the trainee playing the therapist to complete to indicate whether the exercise is too easy or too difficult. Appendix B includes a Deliberate Practice Diary Form that can be used during a training session's final evaluation to process the trainees' experiences, but its primary purpose is to provides trainees a format to explore and record their experiences while engaging in additional, between-session deliberate practice activities without a trainer. Appendix C presents a sample syllabus demonstrating how the 12 deliberate practice exercises and other support material can be integrated into a wider AEDP training course. Instructors may choose to modify the syllabus or pick elements of it to integrate into their own courses.

Downloadable versions of this book's appendixes, including a color version of the Deliberate Practice Reaction Form, can be found in the "Resources" tab at https://www.apa.org/pubs/books/deliberate-practice-accelerated-experiential-dynamic-psychotherapy.

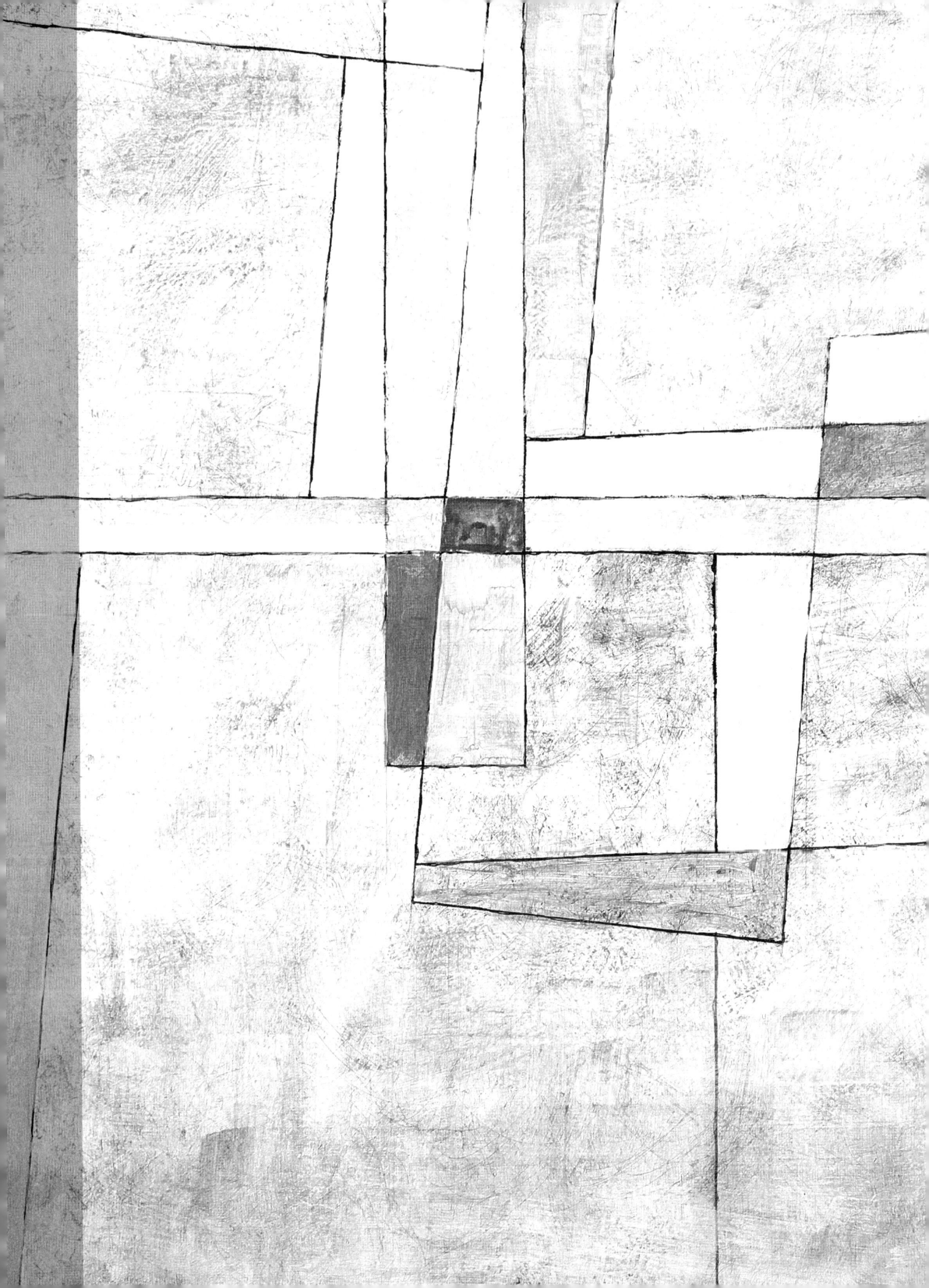

Instructions for the Accelerated Experiential Dynamic Psychotherapy Deliberate Practice Exercises

This chapter provides basic instructions that are common to all the exercises in this book. More specific instructions are provided in each exercise. Chapter 3 also provides important guidance for trainees and trainers that will help them get the most out of deliberate practice. Appendix A offers additional instructions for monitoring and adjusting the difficulty of the exercises as needed after getting through all the client statements in a single difficulty level, including a Deliberate Practice Reaction Form the trainee playing the therapist can complete to indicate whether they found the statements too easy or too difficult. **Difficulty assessment is an important part of the deliberate practice process and should not be skipped.**

Overview

The deliberate practice exercises in this book involve role plays of hypothetical situations in therapy. The role plays involve three people: one trainee role-plays the therapist, another trainee role-plays the client, and a trainer (professor/supervisor) observes and provides feedback. Alternately, a peer can observe and provide feedback.

This book provides a script for each role play, each with a client statement and also with an example therapist response. The client statements are graded in difficulty from beginner to advanced, although these difficulty grades are only estimates. The actual perceived difficulty of client statements is very subjective and varies widely by trainee. For example, some trainees may experience a stimulus of a client being angry as easy to respond to, whereas another trainee may experience it as very difficult. Thus, it is important for trainees to provide difficulty assessments and adjustments to ensure that they are practicing at the right difficulty level: neither too easy nor too hard.

https://doi.org/10.1037/0000439-002

Deliberate Practice in Accelerated Experiential Dynamic Psychotherapy, by N. C. N. Prenn, H. Levenson, A. Vaz, and T. Rousmaniere

Time Frame

We recommend a 90-minute time block for every exercise, structured roughly as follows:

- First 20 minutes: Orientation. The trainer explains the accelerated experiential dynamic psychotherapy (AEDP) skill and demonstrates the exercise procedure with a volunteer trainee.

- Middle 50 minutes: Trainees perform the exercise in pairs. The trainer or a peer provides feedback throughout this process and monitors/adjusts the exercise's difficulty as needed after each set of statements (see Appendix A for more information about difficulty assessment).

- Final 20 minutes: Review, feedback, and discussion.

Preparation

1. Every trainee will need their own copy of this book.

2. Each exercise requires the trainer to fill out a Deliberate Practice Reaction Form after completing all the statements from a single difficulty level. This form is available in the "Resources" tab at https://www.apa.org/pubs/books/deliberate-practice-accelerated-experiential-dynamic-psychotherapy and in Appendix A.

3. Trainees are grouped into pairs. One volunteers to role-play the therapist and one to role-play the client (they will switch roles after 15 minutes of practice). As noted previously, an observer who might be either the trainer or a fellow trainee will work with each pair.

The Role of the Trainer

The primary responsibilities of the trainer are to

1. provide corrective feedback, which includes both information about how well the trainee's response met skill criteria and any necessary guidance about how to improve the response, and

2. remind trainees to do difficulty assessments and adjustments after each level of client statements is completed (beginner, intermediate, and advanced).

How to Practice

Each exercise includes its own step-by-step instructions. Trainees should follow these instructions carefully because every step is important.

Skill Criteria

Each of the first 12 exercises focuses on one essential AEDP skill with one to four skill criteria that describe the important components or principles for that skill.

The goal of the role play is for trainees to practice improvising responses to the client statement in a manner that (a) is attuned to the client, (b) meets skill criteria as closely

as possible, and (c) feels authentic for the trainee. Trainees are provided scripts with example therapist responses to give them a sense of how to incorporate the skill criteria into a response. **It is important, however, that trainees do not read the example responses verbatim in the role plays!** Therapy is highly personal and improvisational; the goal of deliberate practice is to develop trainees' ability to improvise within a consistent framework. Memorizing scripted responses would be counterproductive for helping trainees learn to perform therapy that is responsive, authentic, and attuned to each individual client.

The authors wrote the scripted example responses. However, trainees' personal style of therapy may differ slightly or greatly from that in the example scripts. It is essential that, over time, trainees develop their own style and voice, while simultaneously being able to intervene according to the model's principles and strategies. To facilitate this, the exercises in this book were designed to maximize opportunities for improvisational responses informed by the skill criteria and ongoing feedback.

Review, Feedback, and Discussion

The review and feedback sequence after each role play has these two elements:

- First, the trainee who played the client **briefly** shares how it felt to be on the receiving end of the therapist response. This can help assess how well trainees are attuning with the client.

- Second, the trainer provides **brief** feedback (less than 1 minute) based on the skill criteria for each exercise. Keep feedback specific, behavioral, and brief to preserve time for skill rehearsal. If one trainer is teaching multiple pairs of trainees, the trainer walks around the room, observing the pairs and offering brief feedback. When the trainer is not available, the trainee playing the client gives peer feedback to the therapist, based on the skill criteria and how it felt to be on the receiving end of the intervention. Alternately, a third trainee can observe and provide feedback.

Trainers (or peers) should remember to keep all feedback specific and brief and not to veer into discussions of theory. There are many other settings for extended discussion of AEDP theory and research. In deliberate practice, it is of utmost importance to maximize time for continuous behavioral rehearsal via role plays.

Final Evaluation

After both trainees have role-played the client and the therapist, the trainer provides an evaluation. Participants should engage in a short group discussion based on this evaluation. This discussion can provide ideas for where to focus homework and future deliberate practice sessions. To this end, Appendix B presents a Deliberate Practice Diary Form, which can also be downloaded from the "Resources" tab at https://www.apa.org/pubs/books/deliberate-practice-accelerated-experiential-dynamic-psychotherapy. This form can be used by trainees as part of the final feedback to help trainees process their experiences from that session with the supervisor. However, it is designed primarily to be used as a template for exploring and recording their thoughts and experiences between sessions, particularly when pursuing additional deliberate practice activities without the supervisor, such as rehearsing responses alone or if two trainees want to practice the exercises together, perhaps with a third trainee filling the supervisor's role. Then, if they want, the trainees can discuss these experiences with the supervisor at the beginning of the next training session.

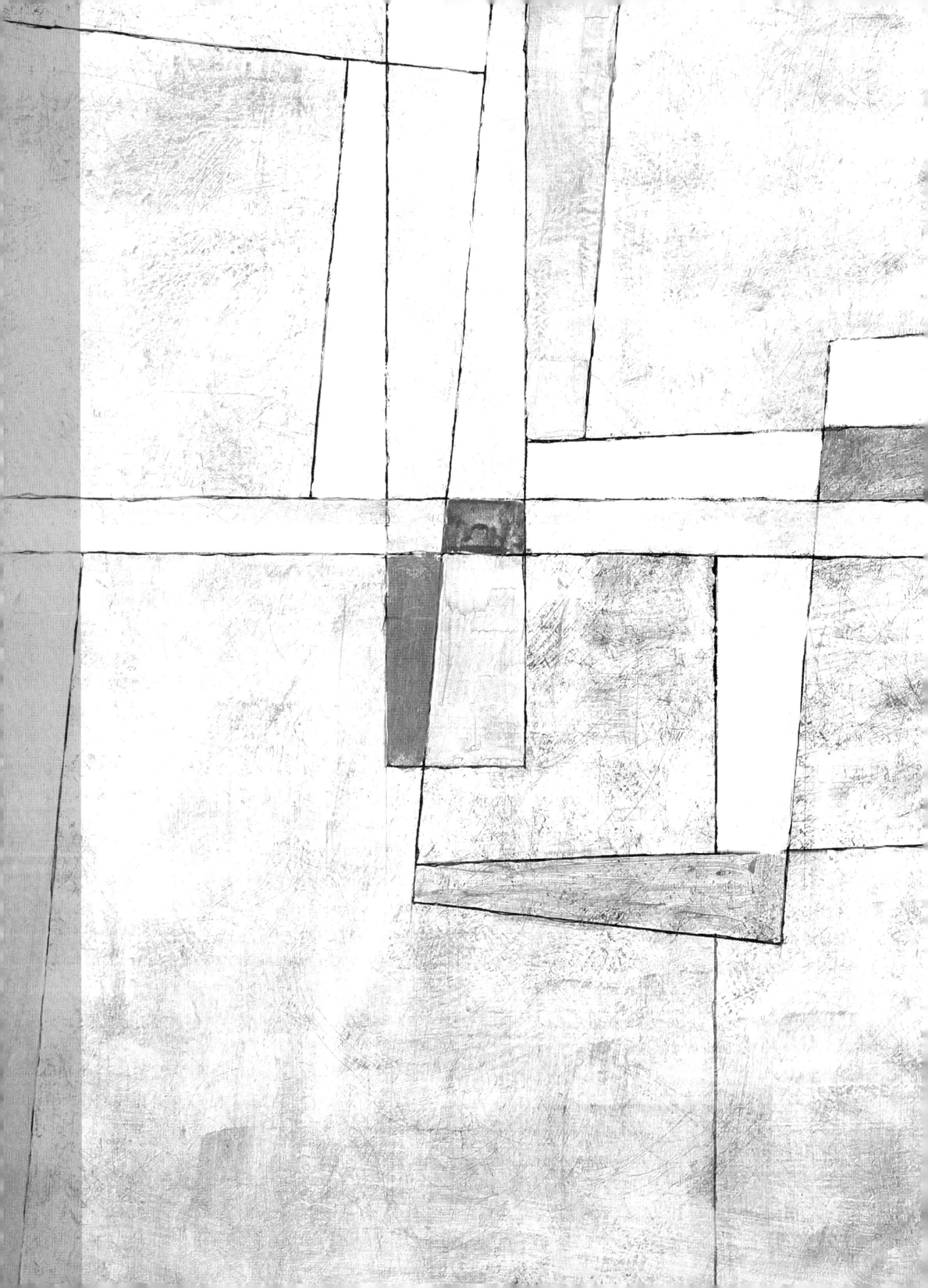

Deliberate Practice Exercises for Accelerated Experiential Dynamic Psychotherapy Skills

This section of the book provides 14 deliberate practice exercises for essential accelerated experiential dynamic psychotherapy (AEDP) skills. These exercises are organized in a developmental sequence, from those that are more appropriate to someone just beginning AEDP training to those who have progressed to a more advanced level. Although we anticipate that most trainers would use these exercises in the order we have suggested, some trainers may find it more appropriate to their training circumstances to use a different order. We also provide two comprehensive exercises that bring together the AEDP skills using an annotated AEDP session transcript and mock AEDP sessions.

Exercises for Beginner Accelerated Experiential Dynamic Psychotherapy Skills

EXERCISE 1: Moment-to-Moment Tracking   25

EXERCISE 2: Exploring and Staying With Physical Experience   37

EXERCISE 3: Undoing Aloneness   53

EXERCISE 4: Affirming   63

Exercises for Intermediate Accelerated Experiential Dynamic Psychotherapy Skills

EXERCISE 5: Self-Involving Self-Disclosure   73

EXERCISE 6: Self-Revealing Self-Disclosure   85

EXERCISE 7: Metaprocessing   95

Exercises for Advanced Accelerated Experiential Dynamic Psychotherapy Skills

EXERCISE 8: Working With Anxiety   107

EXERCISE 9: Affirmative Work With Defenses   119

EXERCISE 10: Initiating Portrayals   131

EXERCISE 11: Privileging Transformance Strivings   143

EXERCISE 12: Metatherapeutic Processing   157

Comprehensive Exercises

EXERCISE 13: Annotated Accelerated Experiential Dynamic Psychotherapy
             Practice Session Transcript   183

EXERCISE 14: Mock Accelerated Experiential Dynamic Psychotherapy Sessions   191

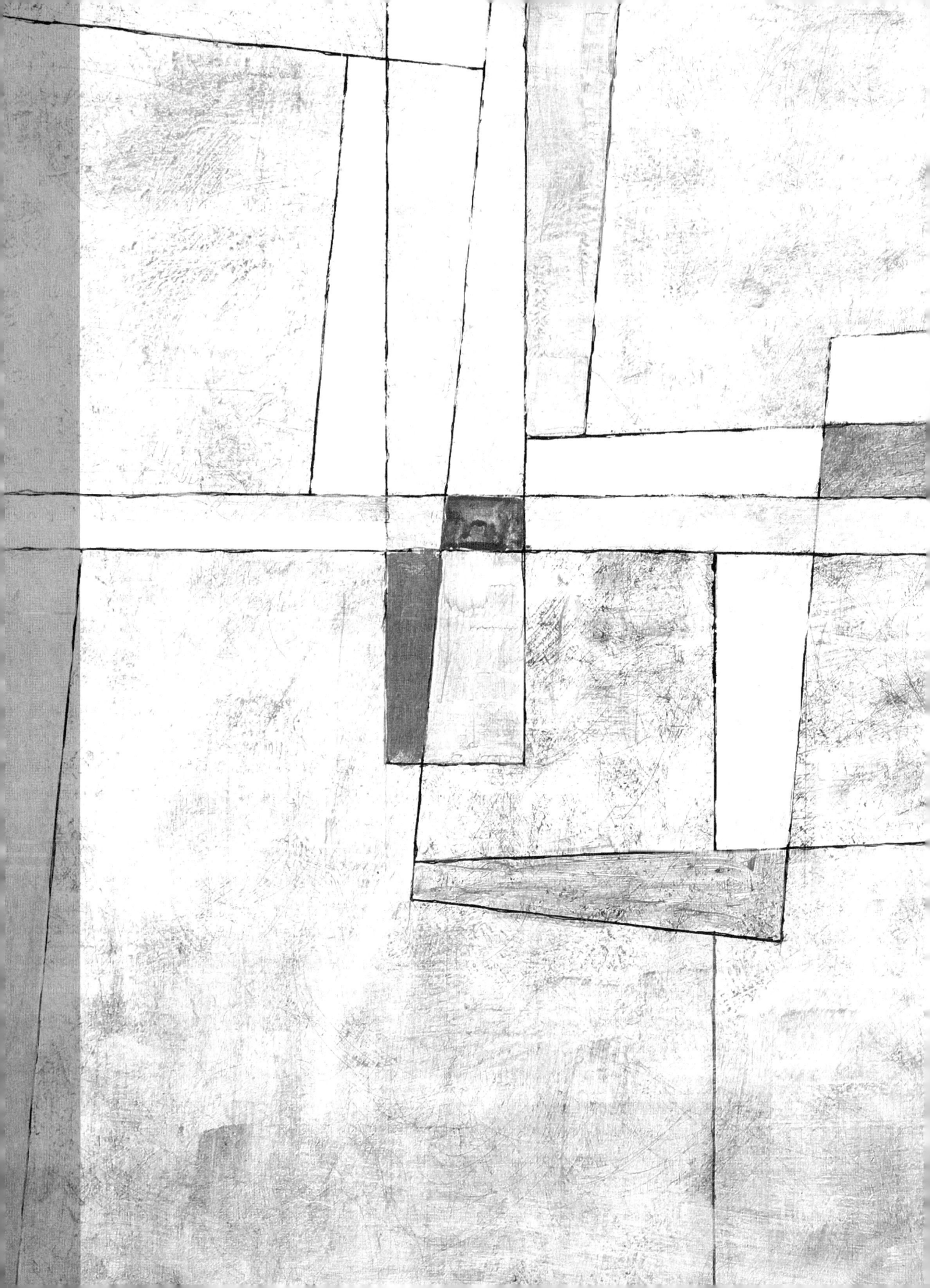

Moment-to-Moment Tracking

Preparations for Exercise 1

1. Read the instructions in Chapter 2.

2. Download the Deliberate Practice Reaction Form and the Deliberate Practice Diary Form at https://www.apa.org/pubs/books/deliberate-practice-accelerated-experiential-dynamic-psychotherapy (see the "Resources" tab; also available in Appendixes A and B, respectively).

Skill Description

Skill Difficulty Level: Beginner

Moment-to-moment tracking is the skill from which all else flows in accelerated-experiential-dynamic-psychotherapy (AEDP). We use moment-to-moment tracking to access, gently and unobtrusively, the here-and-now, body-based experience of the client. Clients are usually unaware that their physical sensations are associated with their emotional reactions. By focusing on how the client's experiences are rooted in the body and being expressed nonverbally, the therapist can help the client be more aware of their internal world.

A large percentage of human communication is nonverbal, and in fact, only a small percentage of communication is conveyed in the language of words themselves. Moment-to-moment tracking is noticing and gently drawing attention to nonverbal, body-based expressions and shifts. Some of these are large movements (e.g., crossing one's arms), and some are micromovements (e.g., a slight wrinkle of the forehead; Hanakawa, 2021).

https://doi.org/10.1037/0000439-003

Deliberate Practice in Accelerated Experiential Dynamic Psychotherapy, by N. C. N. Prenn, H. Levenson, A. Vaz, and T. Rousmaniere

What kinds of things are we tracking? Posture, movement, tension, relaxation, facial expression, shifts in eye contact and gaze direction, speech, tone, volume, pace, congruence, coherence, breathing, and so forth. Why are we tracking? We are tracking physiological reactions and responses because trauma and dynamics are stored in the body and expressed nonverbally.

In a way, one might describe moment-to-moment tracking as interpersonal mindfulness. The therapist does not need to guess or interpret how the client is reacting: All the therapist needs to do is notice and express in body language (mirroring, matching, etc.) and words what they are observing.

In AEDP, we always try to make the implicit experiences that hum along in the background of other therapies explicit; moment-to-moment tracking is a direct route into the implicit.

The therapist's task is to improvise a response to each client statement following this skill criterion: **Name in a statement a nonverbal/physical movement of your client.** Try to keep these short: "You make a fist," "You look away," "Your back straightens," or "Your eyes brighten." This is a deceptively easy-sounding skill, and yet it can be challenging to do because we are so trained to pay attention to the words being spoken.

SKILL CRITERION FOR EXERCISE 1

Name in a statement a nonverbal/physical movement of your client. Make your statement descriptive and short.

HELPFUL HINTS FOR EXERCISE 1

1. As the client, don't worry about "acting" the nonverbals exactly as written. Whatever the actions the therapist sees you are doing will meet the skill criterion as long as the therapist comments on them.

2. The therapist can mirror the client's action, but this is not necessary.

3. As the therapist, be mindful **not** to include interpretations or questions about what the nonverbals mean. This exercise is focused solely on the therapist's tracking what the client is doing moment-to-moment. Of course, when seeing a real client, a therapist will not name every movement the client makes. But here we are isolating one skill and practicing it.

4. As the client, when the therapist's response does not meet criteria, let the therapist know why, rather than just saying, "Let's try it again." Getting good feedback is a critical part of the deliberate practice procedure.

Note: The person playing the client reads the client statement while acting the nonverbal cues presented in brackets.

Examples of Therapists Using Moment-to-Moment Tracking

Example 1

CLIENT: [*Angry*] I'm so angry at my boss! [Start smiling and then look away.]

THERAPIST: You smile and look away.

Example 2

CLIENT: [*Happy*] My vacation with my partner was great. [Let out a big sigh.]

THERAPIST: That's a big sigh.

Example 3

CLIENT: [*Friendly*] I've been coming here for a long time, and I gotta say, I really like being in therapy with you. [Bring your hand up to your mouth, and start biting a nail.]

THERAPIST: Your hand comes to your mouth, and you bite your nail. [The therapist's hand comes up to their mouth, and they start biting a nail.]

INSTRUCTIONS FOR EXERCISE 1

Step 1: Role-Play and Feedback

- The client says the first beginner client statement. The therapist **improvises** a response based on the skill criteria. This exercise works best if the therapist only looks at the client and does not read the client statement.
- The trainer (or, if not available, the client) provides **brief** feedback based on the skill criteria.
- The client then repeats the same statement, and the therapist again improvises a response. The trainer (or client) again provides brief feedback.

Step 2: Repeat

- Repeat Step 1 for all the statements **in the current difficulty level** (beginner, intermediate, or advanced).

Step 3: Assess and Adjust Difficulty

- The therapist completes the Deliberate Practice Reaction Form (see Appendix A) and decides whether to make the exercise easier or harder or to repeat the same difficulty level.

Step 4: Repeat for Approximately 15 Minutes

- Repeat Steps 1 to 3 for at least 15 minutes.
- The trainees then switch therapist and client roles and start over.

Now it's your turn! Follow Steps 1 and 2 from the instructions.

Remember: The goal of the role play is for trainees to practice improvising responses to the client statements in a manner that (a) uses the skill criterion and (b) feels authentic for the trainee. **Example therapist responses for each client statement are provided at the end of this exercise. Trainees should attempt to improvise their own responses before reading the examples.**

   Note: The person playing the client reads the client statement while acting the nonverbal cues presented in brackets. Remember that as the client, you don't have to worry about "acting" the nonverbals exactly as written. Whatever the actions the therapist sees you are doing will meet the skill criterion as long as the therapist comments on them.

BEGINNER CLIENT STATEMENTS FOR EXERCISE 1
Beginner Client Statement 1
[Ashamed] I feel disgusted. [Shake your head.]
Beginner Client Statement 2
[Sad] My mother forgot my birthday. [Smile and look away.]
Beginner Client Statement 3
[Upbeat] I had a great weekend away with my partner. [Stifle a yawn.]
Beginner Client Statement 4
[Depressed] Even getting out of bed is hard. Everything feels like a weight right now. [Rest your chin on your hand.]
Beginner Client Statement 5
[Angry] He's so OCD. It's driving me crazy. [Make a fist.]

 Assess and adjust the difficulty before moving to the next difficulty level (see Step 3 in the exercise instructions).

INTERMEDIATE CLIENT STATEMENTS FOR EXERCISE 1
Intermediate Client Statement 1
[Pressured, talking as fast as you can] I have to find a new job and work is so busy right now and my computer keeps going on the fritz and I need to get to the doctor for my annual physical and my apartment is a mess. [Big exhale.]
Intermediate Client Statement 2
[Confused] I think the most important thing I want you to know is . . . [Stop midsentence.]
Intermediate Client Statement 3
[Sad] I miss him so much. [Close eyes.]
Intermediate Client Statement 4
[Detached/flat] I feel so good and happy. [Stare down at floor.]
Intermediate Client Statement 5
[Disgusted] I really feel like I'm going to throw up. Even thinking about that time makes me have bile at the back of my throat. [Bring hand up to throat.]

 Assess and adjust the difficulty before moving to the next difficulty level (see Step 3 in the exercise instructions).

ADVANCED CLIENT STATEMENTS FOR EXERCISE 1
Advanced Client Statement 1
[Shy] I had a really bad dream. You were in it. [Smile and cover your mouth.]
Advanced Client Statement 2
[Wistful] As you say that, an image of my childhood home comes up; it was such a calm and happy place. Oh, I notice as I say that, my heart starts pounding. [Place hand on your heart.]
Advanced Client Statement 3
[Softly] I really felt good after last week's session. I felt so supported and close to you. I feel embarrassed saying that. [Cover your eyes with your hand.]
Advanced Client Statement 4
[Angry] I wish you hadn't told me that you have children last week. I feel so jealous. [Make a fist.]
Advanced Client Statement 5
[Embarrassed] I feel so much love for you. Is that weird? [Look down.]

 Assess and adjust the difficulty here (see Step 3 in the exercise instructions). If appropriate, follow the instructions to make the exercise even more challenging (see Appendix A).

Example Therapist Responses: Moment-to-Moment Tracking

Remember: Trainees should attempt to improvise their own responses before reading the examples. **Do not read the following responses verbatim unless you are having trouble coming up with your own!**

EXAMPLE RESPONSES TO BEGINNER CLIENT STATEMENTS FOR EXERCISE 1
Example Response to Beginner Client Statement 1
You shake your head as you say that.
Example Response to Beginner Client Statement 2
I notice you smile a bit and look away when you say that.
Example Response to Beginner Client Statement 3
You yawn. [The therapist might yawn too.]
Example Response to Beginner Client Statement 4
You rest your chin on your hand.
Example Response to Beginner Client Statement 5
Your hand makes a fist.

EXAMPLE RESPONSES TO INTERMEDIATE CLIENT STATEMENTS FOR EXERCISE 1
Example Response to Intermediate Client Statement 1
You say that all so fast.
Example Response to Intermediate Client Statement 2
You stopped midsentence.
Example Response to Intermediate Client Statement 3
I see you close your eyes.
Example Response to Intermediate Client Statement 4
You look sad and stare at the floor.
Example Response to Intermediate Client Statement 5
Your hand comes to your throat.

EXAMPLE RESPONSES TO ADVANCED CLIENT STATEMENTS FOR EXERCISE 1
Example Response to Advanced Client Statement 1
Oh, you smile and cover your mouth.
Example Response to Advanced Client Statement 2
One of your hands goes to your heart.
Example Response to Advanced Client Statement 3
You cover your eyes with your hand.
Example Response to Advanced Client Statement 4
You make a fist.
Example Response to Advanced Client Statement 5
You look down as you say that.

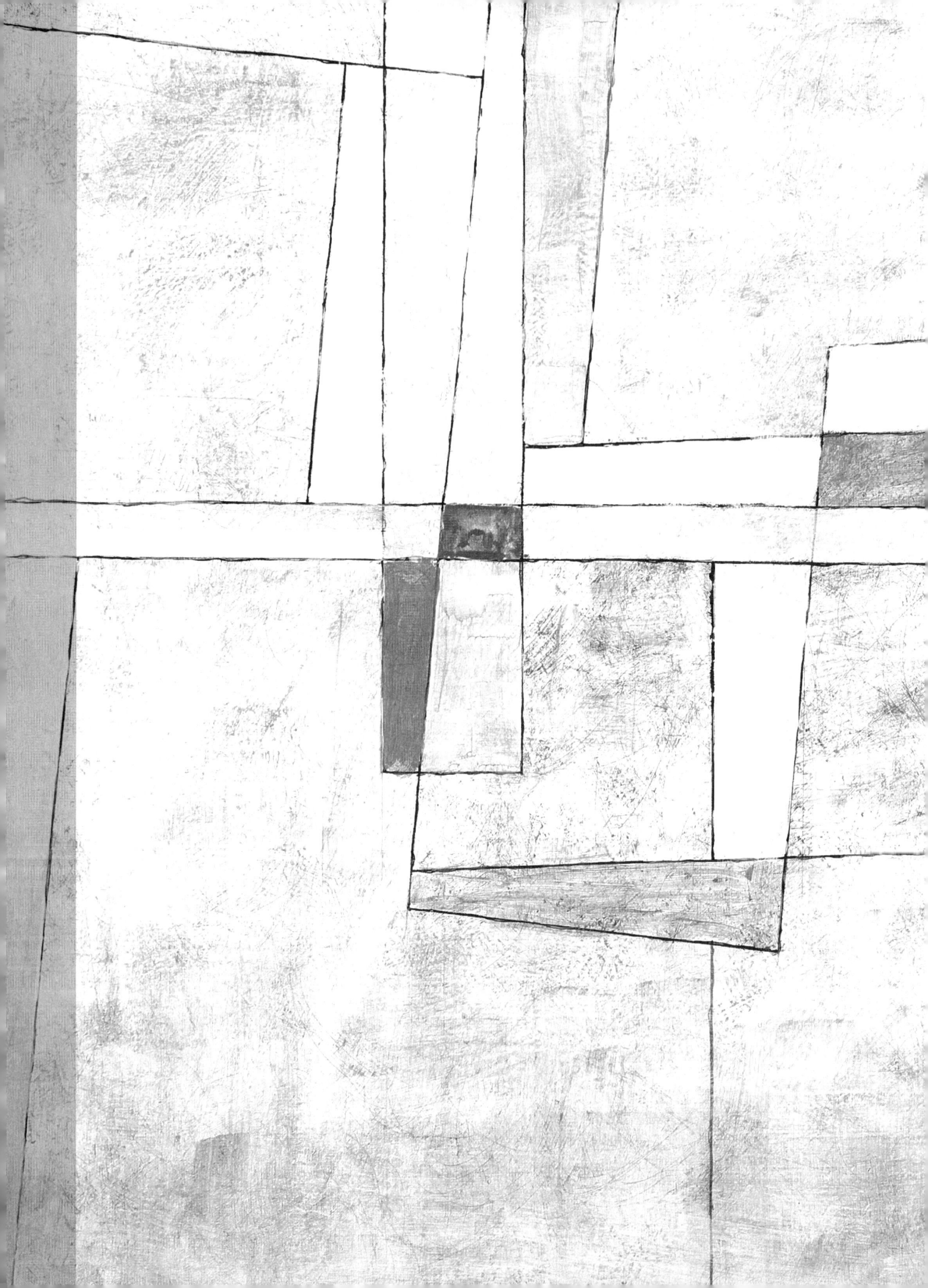

Exploring and Staying With Physical Experience

Preparations for Exercise 2

1. Read the instructions in Chapter 2.

2. Download the Deliberate Practice Reaction Form and the Deliberate Practice Diary Form at https://www.apa.org/pubs/books/deliberate-practice-accelerated-experiential-dynamic-psychotherapy (see the "Resources" tab; also available in Appendixes A and B, respectively).

Skill Description

Skill Difficulty Level: Beginner

In this exercise, we are focusing on two skills that get used so frequently together in accelerated experiential dynamic psychotherapy (AEDP) that we are presenting them as a two-in-one skill package. The first skill is exploring the client's physical experience, and the second is inviting the client to stay with that experience.

When we hear an emotionally evocative word or see an affect-laden gesture or behavior, it provides an entry point into the client's somatic, embodied experience. Inviting the client to get to know how they experience emotions and sensations physically helps clients pay attention to their physical experience and the information emotions give them; it also accesses unprocessed experience, trauma, and somatic memories. Through their moment-to-moment experience, we can access the client's relational and emotional dynamics.

Once we have learned how the client physically experiences something, we like to invite them to stay with that experience. The invitation is literally, "Let's stay with this." The essence of this skill is to help the client experience where they are. The therapist's voice (prosody, intensity, pacing, timbre) can help clients stay with and deepen their experience. Try to use the client's words wherever possible.

https://doi.org/10.1037/0000439-004

Deliberate Practice in Accelerated Experiential Dynamic Psychotherapy, by N. C. N. Prenn, H. Levenson, A. Vaz, and T. Rousmaniere

The therapist's task is to improvise a response to each client statement following these skill criteria:

1. **Notice an affect-laden word or sentence and invite the client to describe their physical experience.** "How do you experience that physically?" is a relatively neutral way to ask about somatic experience. After making this invitation, wait for the person playing the client to reply with their scripted statement. Then proceed to the next skill criterion.

2. **Explicitly ask if the two of you can stay with the client's experience.** Ask the client to stay with experience. Neither you nor the client needs to try to figure out or have a pre-conceived idea of what the somatic experience means—the skill is just to stay with it.

Note: Because we are asking the client two questions, the format follows a dialogue procedure.

SKILL CRITERIA FOR EXERCISE 2

1. Notice an affect-laden word and invite the client to describe their physical experience.
2. Explicitly ask if the two of you can stay with the client's experience.

Examples of Therapists Exploring and Staying With Physical Experiences

Example 1

CLIENT: [*Sad*] I'm so sad about my dog dying.

THERAPIST: Oh my . . . how do you experience the sadness physically? (Criterion 1)

CLIENT: It's like a sharp pain in my heart.

THERAPIST: Can we just stay with the feeling of the sharp pain in your heart? (Criterion 2)

Example 2

CLIENT: [*Scared*] No one's here to help me.

THERAPIST: And what is that like—the physical feeling that there is no one here to help you? (Criterion 1)

CLIENT: It's a tightness in my chest right here. (Puts hand on ribs)

THERAPIST: Can we just stay with the tightness in your chest? (Putting hand on ribs) (Criterion 2)

Example 3

CLIENT: [*Proud*] I can't believe I was finally able to stand up to my boss!

THERAPIST: And when you stood up to your boss, what did that feel like in your body? (Criterion 2)

CLIENT: It felt like powerful energy.

THERAPIST: [*Smiling broadly*] Wow! Can we stay with that feeling of powerful energy? (Criterion 2)

INSTRUCTIONS FOR EXERCISE 2

Step 1: Role-Play and Feedback

- The client initiates the dialogue by reading the first statement in the initial beginner dialogue. The therapist **improvises** a response following the first skill criterion.
- The supervisor (or, if not available, the client) provides **brief** feedback based on the skill criterion. If the criterion was not met, the client repeats the same statement, and the therapist again improvises responses until it is easy to meet the skill criterion.
- The patient then reads the next statement in the same dialogue, and the therapist responds using the second criterion.
- The supervisor again provides feedback and repeats the second statement until the therapist meets the skill criterion.

Step 2: Repeat

- Repeat Step 1 for all the dialogues **in the current difficulty level** (beginner, intermediate, or advanced).

Step 3: Assess and Adjust Difficulty

- The therapist completes the Deliberate Practice Reaction Form (see Appendix A) and decides whether to make the exercise easier or harder or to repeat the same difficulty level.

Step 4: Repeat for Approximately 15 Minutes

- Repeat Steps 1 to 3 for at least 15 minutes.
- The trainees then switch therapist and client roles and start over.

➡️ **Now it's your turn! Follow Steps 1 and 2 from the instructions.**

Remember: The goal of the role play is for trainees to practice improvising responses to the client statements in a manner that (a) uses the skill criteria and (b) feels authentic for the trainee. **Example therapist responses for each client statement are provided at the end of this exercise. Trainees should attempt to improvise their own responses before reading the examples.**

BEGINNER DIALOGUE 1
CLIENT: **[Sad]** I have felt so alone my whole life.
THERAPIST PROMPT (CRITERION 1): Invite the client to describe their physical experience.
CLIENT: **[Sadder]** It is like a black cloud coming down over my eyes.
THERAPIST PROMPT (CRITERION 2): Explicitly ask if the two of you can stay with the client's experience.

BEGINNER DIALOGUE 2
CLIENT: **[Open]** Last week's session made me feel hopeful that I can get better.
THERAPIST PROMPT (CRITERION 1): Invite the client to describe their physical experience.
CLIENT: **[Calm]** It was oddly warm in my heart and felt comforting.
THERAPIST PROMPT (CRITERION 2): Explicitly ask if the two of you can stay with the client's experience.

BEGINNER DIALOGUE 3
CLIENT: [Thoughtful] I am missing my parents so much.
THERAPIST PROMPT (CRITERION 1): Invite the client to describe their physical experience.
CLIENT: [Sad] It is a pain in my chest.
THERAPIST PROMPT (CRITERION 2): Explicitly ask if the two of you can stay with the client's experience.

BEGINNER DIALOGUE 4
CLIENT: [Downcast] Even when I am with other people, I feel alone and like I have a wall up. Does that make sense?
THERAPIST PROMPT (CRITERION 1): Invite the client to describe their physical experience.
CLIENT: [Sad] My heart feels hard and impenetrable.
THERAPIST PROMPT (CRITERION 2): Explicitly ask if the two of you can stay with the client's experience.

BEGINNER DIALOGUE 5
CLIENT: [Shaking head and smiling] I had such a good time at the party. I didn't expect to. I felt like myself and that I fit in with everyone.
THERAPIST PROMPT (CRITERION 1): Invite the client to describe their physical experience.
CLIENT: [Interested] It's like I have energy coming up inside of me in all different directions.
THERAPIST PROMPT (CRITERION 2): Explicitly ask if the two of you can stay with the client's experience.

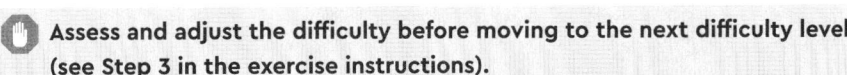 **Assess and adjust the difficulty before moving to the next difficulty level (see Step 3 in the exercise instructions).**

INTERMEDIATE DIALOGUE 1
CLIENT: [**Nod and smile**] I felt so grateful. My friend reaching out to me meant a lot.
THERAPIST PROMPT (CRITERION 1): Invite the client to describe their physical experience.
CLIENT: [**Smiling**] It feels warm and emotional.
THERAPIST PROMPT (CRITERION 2): Explicitly ask if the two of you can stay with the client's experience.

INTERMEDIATE DIALOGUE 2
CLIENT: [**Pressured speech**] My anxiety overwhelms me inside. Sometimes I can't even hear what other people are saying. I have so many thoughts coming all at once. I feel completely overwhelmed. I can't get anything done.
THERAPIST PROMPT (CRITERION 1): Invite the client to describe their physical experience.
CLIENT: [**Sad**] My heart is racing and it feels hard to breathe.
THERAPIST PROMPT (CRITERION 2): Explicitly ask if the two of you can stay with the client's experience.

INTERMEDIATE DIALOGUE 3
CLIENT: [**Flat and weary**] I feel so down. I've been isolating. Friends keep texting and reaching out, but I don't reply.
THERAPIST PROMPT (CRITERION 1): Invite the client to describe their physical experience.
CLIENT: [**Sadder**] It is hollow and heavy all in my belly.
THERAPIST PROMPT (CRITERION 2): Explicitly ask if the two of you can stay with the client's experience.

INTERMEDIATE DIALOGUE 4
CLIENT: [Frustrated] I was at my meditation circle on Zoom last night. These are all my friends. They all seemed to be feeling connected, yet I felt like such an outsider.
THERAPIST PROMPT (CRITERION 1): Invite the client to describe their physical experience.
CLIENT: [Sad] It's so familiar—like a black curtain comes down over me and my face feels blank and frozen.
THERAPIST PROMPT (CRITERION 2): Explicitly ask if the two of you can stay with the client's experience.

INTERMEDIATE DIALOGUE 5
CLIENT: [Eager] Wow. I feel like I'm just reporting to you. Where should we be?
THERAPIST PROMPT (CRITERION 1): Invite the client to describe their physical experience.
CLIENT: [Sad] It's like my body is floating in a drifty sort of way.
THERAPIST PROMPT (CRITERION 2): Explicitly ask if the two of you can stay with the client's experience.

 Assess and adjust the difficulty before moving to the next difficulty level (see Step 3 in the exercise instructions).

ADVANCED DIALOGUE 1

CLIENT: [Fearful] I'm not scared of my feelings, but I am scared of this pain that's coming up. It feels like I'm going to panic and so I fight it. I don't want it to come back.
THERAPIST PROMPT (CRITERION 1): Invite the client to describe their physical experience.
CLIENT: [Sad] It feels like a lump with spikes coming out of it.
THERAPIST PROMPT (CRITERION 2): Explicitly ask if the two of you can stay with the client's experience.

ADVANCED DIALOGUE 2

CLIENT: [Tired] I feel like I am torturing myself with all the things I've ever done that I feel bad about. I'm feeling so guilty imagining all the people that I have hurt.
THERAPIST PROMPT (CRITERION 1): Invite the client to describe their physical experience.
CLIENT: [Slumped over] It's like my stomach is lurching.
THERAPIST PROMPT (CRITERION 2): Explicitly ask if the two of you can stay with the client's experience.

ADVANCED DIALOGUE 3

CLIENT: [Frustrated] I want to connect with him so badly. He keeps shutting me out. He says he's there for me, but I don't trust that. I feel so frustrated.
THERAPIST PROMPT (CRITERION 1): Invite the client to describe their physical experience.
CLIENT: [More frustrated] It is like the center of my chest is a ball of rage.
THERAPIST PROMPT (CRITERION 2): Explicitly ask if the two of you can stay with the client's experience.

ADVANCED DIALOGUE 4
CLIENT: [Hopeless] When she gives me that look, I know what she is thinking. I don't even think she likes me anymore.
THERAPIST PROMPT (CRITERION 1): Invite the client to describe their physical experience.
CLIENT: [Slumped over] It feels like I'm small, like I am actually shrinking in size.
THERAPIST PROMPT (CRITERION 2): Explicitly ask if the two of you can stay with the client's experience.

ADVANCED DIALOGUE 5
CLIENT: [Staring into space] I can feel myself numbing out and spacing out. I almost feel dizzy.
THERAPIST PROMPT (CRITERION 1): Invite the client to describe their physical experience.
CLIENT: [More frustrated] It feels like a swirling in my head and a weird blankness.
THERAPIST PROMPT (CRITERION 2): Explicitly ask if the two of you can stay with the client's experience.

 Assess and adjust the difficulty here (see Step 3 in the exercise instructions). If appropriate, follow the instructions to make the exercise even more challenging (see Appendix A).

Example Therapist Responses: Exploring and Staying With Physical Experiences

Remember: Trainees should attempt to improvise their own responses before reading the examples. **Do not read the following responses verbatim unless you are having trouble coming up with your own!**

EXAMPLE THERAPIST RESPONSES FOR BEGINNER DIALOGUE 1
CLIENT: [Sad] I have felt so alone my whole life.
THERAPIST: And what is that like inside physically?
CLIENT: [Sadder] It is like a black cloud coming down over my eyes.
THERAPIST: Would it be okay with you if we stayed with the black cloud coming down over your eyes?

EXAMPLE THERAPIST RESPONSES FOR BEGINNER DIALOGUE 2
CLIENT: [Open] Last week's session made me feel hopeful that I can get better
THERAPIST: What was that like inside?
CLIENT: [Calm] It was oddly warm in my heart and felt comforting.
THERAPIST: Can we stay with that feeling of oddly warm in your heart and comforting?

EXAMPLE THERAPIST RESPONSES FOR BEGINNER DIALOGUE 3
CLIENT: [Thoughtful] I am missing my parents so much.
THERAPIST: What does the missing feel like on the inside?
CLIENT: [Sad] It is a pain in my chest.
THERAPIST: Would it be okay with you if we stayed with the pain in your chest?

EXAMPLE THERAPIST RESPONSES FOR BEGINNER DIALOGUE 4
CLIENT: [Downcast] Even when I am with other people, I feel alone and like I have a wall up. Does that make sense?
THERAPIST: Yes, it does make sense. And what is that wall like inside physically?
CLIENT: [Sad] My heart feels hard and impenetrable.
THERAPIST: Would it be okay with you if we stayed with the hard and impenetrable sense of your heart and get to know it?

EXAMPLE THERAPIST RESPONSES FOR BEGINNER DIALOGUE 5
CLIENT: [Shaking head and smiling] I had such a good time at the party. I didn't expect to. I felt like myself and that I fit in with everyone.
THERAPIST: What's it like inside that you felt like yourself?
CLIENT: [Interested] It is like I have energy coming up inside of me in all different directions.
THERAPIST: Would it be okay with you if we stay with that energy inside of you?

EXAMPLE THERAPIST RESPONSES FOR INTERMEDIATE DIALOGUE 1

CLIENT: [Nod and smile] I felt so grateful. My friend reaching out to me meant a lot.
THERAPIST: What is the grateful like inside?
CLIENT: [Smiling] It feels warm and emotional.
THERAPIST: Would it be okay for us to stay with the warm emotional feeling?

EXAMPLE THERAPIST RESPONSES FOR INTERMEDIATE DIALOGUE 2

CLIENT: [Pressured speech] My anxiety overwhelms me inside. Sometimes I can't even hear what other people are saying. I have so many thoughts coming all at once. I feel completely overwhelmed. I can't get anything done.
THERAPIST: Walk me into your experience of being overwhelmed. What is that like inside?
CLIENT: [Wide eyed] My heart is racing and it feels hard to breathe.
THERAPIST: Would it be okay with you if we stayed with your racing heart and feeling of hard to breathe?

EXAMPLE THERAPIST RESPONSES FOR INTERMEDIATE DIALOGUE 3

CLIENT: [Flat and weary] I feel so down. I have been isolating. Friends keep texting and reaching out, but I don't respond.
THERAPIST: And what is that like inside the down feeling?
CLIENT: [Sadder] It is hollow and heavy all in my belly.
THERAPIST: [Putting hand on belly] Would it be okay with you if we stayed with that hollow and heavy all in your belly feeling?

EXAMPLE THERAPIST RESPONSES FOR INTERMEDIATE DIALOGUE 4
CLIENT: [Frustrated] I was at my meditation circle on Zoom last night. These are all my friends. They all seemed to be feeling connected, yet I felt like such an outsider.
THERAPIST: And what is that like inside the feeling like such an outsider?
CLIENT: [Sad] It's so familiar—like a black curtain comes down over me and my face feels blank and frozen.
THERAPIST: Would it be okay with you if we stayed with that feeling of a black curtain coming down and your face feeling blank and frozen?

EXAMPLE THERAPIST RESPONSES FOR INTERMEDIATE DIALOGUE 5
CLIENT: [Eager] Wow. I feel like I'm just reporting to you. Where should we be?
THERAPIST: What's it like inside the feeling of just reporting?
CLIENT: [Sad] It's like my body is floating in a drifty sort of way.
THERAPIST: Would it be okay with you if we stayed with that sort of floating, drifty feeling?

EXAMPLE THERAPIST RESPONSES FOR ADVANCED DIALOGUE 1

CLIENT: **[Fearful]** I'm not scared of my feelings, but I am scared of this pain that's coming up. It feels like I'm going to panic and so I fight it. I don't want it to come back.

THERAPIST: What does that feel like physically—this pain that's coming up?

CLIENT: **[Sad]** It feels like a hard lump with spikes coming out of it.

THERAPIST: Would it be okay with you if we stayed with that hard lump with spikes coming out of it?

EXAMPLE THERAPIST RESPONSES FOR ADVANCED DIALOGUE 2

CLIENT: **[Tired]** I feel like I am torturing myself with all the things I've ever done that I feel bad about. I'm feeling so guilty imagining all the people that I have hurt.

THERAPIST: And what does that guilt feel like in your body?

CLIENT: **[Slumped over]** It's like my stomach is lurching.

THERAPIST: Would it be okay with you if we stayed with the physical feeling of your stomach's lurching?

EXAMPLE THERAPIST RESPONSES FOR ADVANCED DIALOGUE 3

CLIENT: **[Frustrated]** I want to connect with him so badly. He keeps shutting me out. He says he's there for me, but I don't trust that. I feel so frustrated.

THERAPIST: What's that like physically the frustration?

CLIENT: **[More frustrated]** It is like a ball of rage.

THERAPIST: Would it be okay with you if we stayed with that ball of rage?

EXAMPLE THERAPIST RESPONSES FOR ADVANCED DIALOGUE 4
CLIENT: **[Hopeless]** When she gives me that look, I know what she is thinking. I don't even think she likes me anymore.
THERAPIST: What does that feel like in your body when she gives you that look?
CLIENT: **[Slumped over]** It feels like I'm small and like I am actually shrinking in size.
THERAPIST: Would it be okay with you if we stayed with that small, shrinking in size feeling?

EXAMPLE THERAPIST RESPONSES FOR ADVANCED DIALOGUE 5
CLIENT: **[Staring into space]** I can feel myself numbing out and spacing out. I almost feel dizzy.
THERAPIST: What's that like inside that numbing, almost dizzy feeling?
CLIENT: **[Frowning with concentration]** It feels like a swirling in my head and a weird blankness.
THERAPIST: Would it be okay with you if we lingered with that swirling in your head, weird blankness and got to know it?

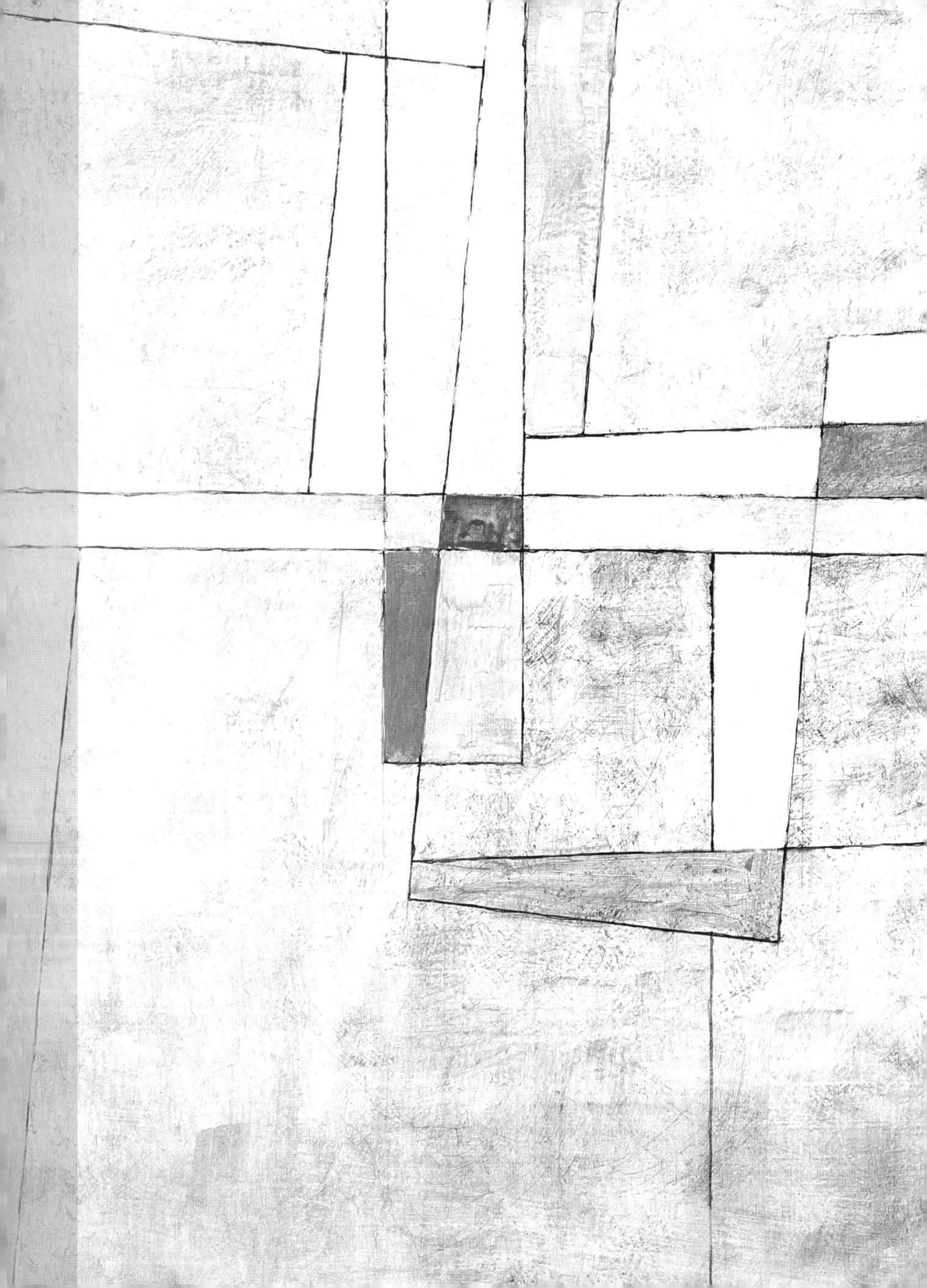

Undoing Aloneness

Preparations for Exercise 3

1. Read the instructions in Chapter 2.

2. Download the Deliberate Practice Reaction Form and the Deliberate Practice Diary Form at https://www.apa.org/pubs/books/deliberate-practice-accelerated-experiential-dynamic-psychotherapy (see the "Resources" tab; also available in Appendixes A and B, respectively).

Skill Description

Skill Difficulty Level: Beginner

Accelerated experiential dynamic psychotherapy (AEDP) understands psychopathology to result from the client's "unwilled and unwanted aloneness" in the face of overwhelming or painful emotional experiences (Fosha, 2009, p. 182). Undoing aloneness is a critical skill in AEDP. It is the goal of the therapist to make explicit that they are with the client. We do this in three ways: (a) with our body language and paraverbals; (b) by using "we" language and by saying and making explicit that we, the therapist, are with the client; and (c) by explicitly inquiring about the client–therapist connection and client's sense of the therapist's presence. We do not assume that a client feels our presence; we ask to make it explicit.

A tenet of AEDP is that we hold a client "in our heart and mind." This means that we remember details about clients and let them know that we know them and remember the things they tell us about their lives. For example, "Yes, I remember your friend, Amal. You told me about her a few weeks ago." What keeps these interventions safe and rigorous is that they are always metaprocessed—a skill you will practice in Exercise 7—with the therapist's exploring how the client is responding to them in real time. "What is it like that I do remember your friend?"

https://doi.org/10.1037/0000439-005

Deliberate Practice in Accelerated Experiential Dynamic Psychotherapy, by N. C. N. Prenn, H. Levenson, A. Vaz, and T. Rousmaniere

The therapist should improvise a response to each client statement following these skill criteria:

1. **Use paraverbal and nonverbal behaviors to reinforce your presence.** Nonverbals (e.g., nodding, leaning in, putting hand to heart, a clap), paraverbals (e.g., mmming, wincing, sighing, a-ha-ing), and barely verbals (e.g., ya, right, yup, ouch) make up a large percentage of interventions in AEDP.

2. **State or use words that imply you are present with the client.** In AEDP we make the relationship explicit. We use statements such as "I am here with you," "You are not alone," "Feel me with you." In addition, we use psychoeducational statements: "It is important that you feel me with you; you've been alone with this too much." Using words that imply you are present, such as "share" and "with," remind the client that you are alongside them (e.g., "I am smiling with you").

3. **Ask or invite the client to take in your presence.** For example, the standard undoing aloneness question is "Can you feel me with you?" This is an additional level of work (and therefore, awareness) for the client to reflect on whether they can feel the therapist's presence and respond to the question, furthering the likelihood that the client's sense of aloneness will be alleviated. If the client is having difficulty letting in your presence, you can use that information to focus the work on building the client's receptive affective and relational capacities.

SKILL CRITERIA FOR EXERCISE 3

1. Use paraverbal and nonverbal behaviors to reinforce your presence.
2. State or use words that imply you are present with the client.
3. Ask or invite the client to take in your presence.

Examples of Therapists Undoing Aloneness

Example 1

CLIENT: [*Sad*] I'm so sad about my dog dying.

THERAPIST: Ooh. [Leaning forward] (Criterion 1) I'm here with you, and my heart aches for your loss. (Criterion 2) Can you feel me with you right now? (Criterion 3)

Example 2

CLIENT: [*Scared*] I'm all alone. No one's here to help me.

THERAPIST: [Leaning forward] (Criterion 1) I am here and would like to help. (Criterion 2) Would it be okay to check in to be sure you feel me here with you? (Criterion 3)

Example 3

CLIENT: [*Proud*] I can't believe I was finally able to stand up to my boss!

THERAPIST: [Broad smile] (Criterion 1) I'm so excited with you! (Criterion 2) What's it like for me to share in this pride with you? (Criterion 3)

INSTRUCTIONS FOR EXERCISE 3

Step 1: Role-Play and Feedback

- The client says the first beginner client statement. The therapist **improvises** a response based on the skill criteria.
- The trainer (or, if not available, the client) provides **brief** feedback based on the skill criteria.
- The client then repeats the same statement, and the therapist again improvises a response. The trainer (or client) again provides brief feedback.

Step 2: Repeat

- Repeat Step 1 for all the statements **in the current difficulty level** (beginner, intermediate, or advanced).

Step 3: Assess and Adjust Difficulty

- The therapist completes the Deliberate Practice Reaction Form (see Appendix A) and decides whether to make the exercise easier or harder or to repeat the same difficulty level.

Step 4: Repeat for Approximately 15 Minutes

- Repeat Steps 1 to 3 for at least 15 minutes.
- The trainees then switch therapist and client roles and start over.

⮕ **Now it's your turn! Follow Steps 1 and 2 from the instructions.**

Remember: The goal of the role play is for trainees to practice improvising responses to the client statements in a manner that (a) uses the skill criteria and (b) feels authentic for the trainee. **Example therapist responses for each client statement are provided at the end of this exercise. Trainees should attempt to improvise their own responses before reading the examples.**

BEGINNER CLIENT STATEMENTS FOR EXERCISE 3
Beginner Client Statement 1
[Sad] I have felt so lonely and alone my whole life.
Beginner Client Statement 2
[Yearning] As a little boy I would walk past houses on my street and make up stories of living with those happy families.
Beginner Client Statement 3
[Thoughtful] I have butterflies in my stomach as I'm talking. I feel nervous, I guess. I'm not sure why.
Beginner Client Statement 4
[Sad] Even when I am with other people I feel alone and like I have a wall up. Does that make sense?
Beginner Client Statement 5
[Unsure] I feel like I am talking to myself. I just wanted you to get the context of all of that, I guess.

✋ **Assess and adjust the difficulty before moving to the next difficulty level (see Step 3 in the exercise instructions).**

INTERMEDIATE CLIENT STATEMENTS FOR EXERCISE 3
Intermediate Client Statement 1
[Pleased and surprised] No one has ever noticed that I hold my breath like that.
Intermediate Client Statement 2
[Leg bouncing] My anxiety overwhelms me inside. Sometimes I can't even hear what other people are saying. I have so many thoughts coming all at once.
Intermediate Client Statement 3
[Sad] I feel so down. I've been isolating. Friends keep texting and reaching out, but I don't respond.
Intermediate Client Statement 4
[Downcast] I was at my meditation circle last night. These are all my friends. They all seemed to be feeling connected, yet I felt like such an outsider.
Intermediate Client Statement 5
[Thoughtful] I feel like I am just reporting to you. Where should we be?

 Assess and adjust the difficulty before moving to the next difficulty level (see Step 3 in the exercise instructions).

ADVANCED CLIENT STATEMENTS FOR EXERCISE 3
Advanced Client Statement 1
[Eyes wide with fear] I'm not scared of my feelings, but I am scared of this pain that comes up. It feels like I'm going to panic and so I fight it. I don't want it to come back.
Advanced Client Statement 2
[Frustrated] I can't sleep. I'm awake all night long. I feel like I am torturing myself with all the things I've ever done that I feel bad about.
Advanced Client Statement 3
[Desolate] I want to connect with him so badly. He keeps shutting me out. He says he's there for me, but I don't trust that. He has said that before.
Advanced Client Statement 4
[Shaking head in confusion] When they give me that look, I know what they are thinking. I don't even think they like me anymore.
Advanced Client Statement 5
[Blankly] I can feel myself numbing out and spacing out. I almost feel dizzy.

✋ **Assess and adjust the difficulty here (see Step 3 in the exercise instructions). If appropriate, follow the instructions to make the exercise even more challenging (see Appendix A).**

Example Therapist Responses: Undoing Aloneness

Remember: Trainees should attempt to improvise their own responses before reading the examples. **Do not read the following responses verbatim unless you are having trouble coming up with your own!**

EXAMPLE RESPONSES TO BEGINNER CLIENT STATEMENTS FOR EXERCISE 3
Example Response to Beginner Client Statement 1
Oh, ow. (Criterion 1) I am here with you. (Criterion 2) Let yourself experience me with you, if you can. (Criterion 3)
Example Response to Beginner Client Statement 2
[Leaning forward] (Criterion 1) What a lonely feeling. The most important thing for us is that you feel me with you right now. (Criterion 2) Do you sense my presence? (Criterion 3)
Example Response to Beginner Client Statement 3
[Soft voice] (Criterion 1) I'm here with you. (Criterion 2) Right now as you're talking, can you feel me with you? (Criterion 3)
Example Response to Beginner Client Statement 4
[Leaning forward] (Criterion 1) As I am here with you, it makes perfect sense to me. (Criterion 2) Can you feel me with you right now or do you have that wall up with me too? (Criterion 3)
Example Response to Beginner Client Statement 5
[Looking into the eyes of the client] (Criterion 1) As I am sitting here with you, I feel everything you are saying is so important and I want to hear it all. (Criterion 2) And, would it be okay for just right now to let yourself feel me with you? (Criterion 3)

EXAMPLE RESPONSES TO INTERMEDIATE CLIENT STATEMENTS FOR EXERCISE 3

Example Response to Intermediate Client Statement 1

[Nodding and mmming] (Criterion 1) I am here noticing. Feel me with you. (Criterion 2) Do you have a sense of me with you? (Criterion 3)

Example Response to Intermediate Client Statement 2

[Nods and makes eye contact] (Criterion 1) I am so glad you are telling me. I'm here. (Criterion 2) So the most important thing right now is to take a breath and feel if you can get a sense of me with you (Criterion 3) and ask the thoughts to give us some space to be together.

Example Response to Intermediate Client Statement 3

[Smiles and leans forward] (Criterion 1) So right here right now with me . . . this may seem like an odd question, do you feel me with you? (Criterion 3) It's important you don't feel alone while you're here with me. (Criterion 2)

Example Response to Intermediate Client Statement 4

[With feeling and pain] Oh! (Criterion 1) What a hard feeling. (Criterion 2) So right here with me, do you feel connected to me? (Criterion 3)

Example Response to Intermediate Client Statement 5

[Big smile and nodding head] (Criterion 1) You are doing great. It's important to know what is going on, and the most important thing is that we make sure you feel me alongside you (Criterion 2) as you're talking. Do you have a sense of me? (Criterion 3)

EXAMPLE RESPONSES TO ADVANCED CLIENT STATEMENTS FOR EXERCISE 3

Example Response to Advanced Client Statement 1

[Hand to heart, wrinkling forehead] (Criterion 1) I get how scary the pain and feeling of panic can be and the most important thing is that you're not alone with it. (Criterion 2) Let's both put our feet on the ground and work on our connection together . . . would it be okay to try to help you feel less alone with this? (Criterion 3)

Example Response to Advanced Client Statement 2

[Wincing] Oooh! (Criterion 1) That is such a lonely experience. Feel me with you right now, (Criterion 2) and let's work on you really taking me in (Criterion 3) so that over time you'll feel less alone when you're awake at night.

Example Response to Advanced Client Statement 3

[Making a serious confident face] (Criterion 1) So you are right here with me. This may sound like a funny question, but do you feel me wanting to be there for you? (Criterion 3) I get how hard it is to trust when you've been hurt by him, and I'm wanting to see if we can look at this together. (Criterion 2)

Example Response to Advanced Client Statement 4

Oh, mmm. (Criterion 1) I don't want you alone with this feeling. (Criterion 2) Can we check in on how connected you feel with me as you're talking? (Criterion 3)

Example Response to Advanced Client Statement 5

[Nodding and with soft eyes making eye contact gently using slow voice] (Criterion 1) I'm here with you. (Criterion 2) Let yourself come back to us if you can, and if not, that's okay. Let's just slowly and gently try to reconnect with yourself and me (Criterion 3)—let your eyes look at mine if they can.

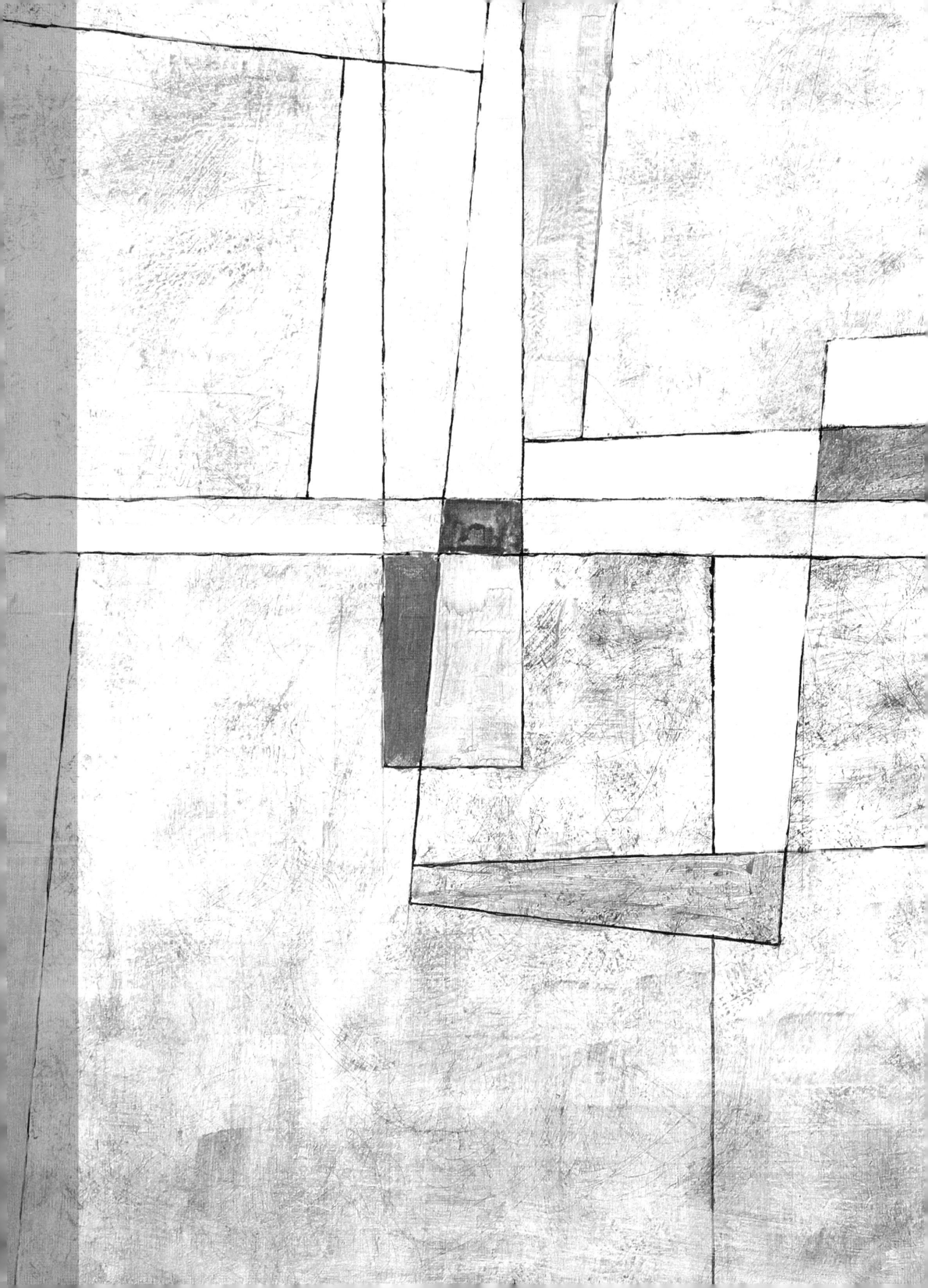

Affirming

Preparations for Exercise 4

1. Read the instructions in Chapter 2.

2. Download the Deliberate Practice Reaction Form and the Deliberate Practice Diary Form at https://www.apa.org/pubs/books/deliberate-practice-accelerated-experiential-dynamic-psychotherapy (see the "Resources" tab; also available in Appendixes A and B, respectively).

Skill Description

Skill Difficulty Level: Beginner

It is important as we introduce the skill of affirming to make explicit that although accelerated experiential dynamic psychotherapy (AEDP), like most other forms of therapy, deals with pain, trauma, and suffering, the AEDP therapist works to have the therapy and the therapeutic relationship feel good. Affirming is one of the interventions that sets this in motion. The AEDP therapist is supportive, validating, and emotionally engaged from the first moments of the first session and throughout the therapy. Affirming is an intervention that promotes safety and trust by acknowledging and validating the client's experiences, strengths, and emotions. Above all else, the therapist's affirming and supporting explicitly and specifically all that a client is clearly doing in therapy, translates into building confidence in clients that their experiences make sense and that they are doing therapy right. All of this sets off a positive chain reaction of physiological responses including the release of the neurotransmitter dopamine and its concomitant increase in motivation, improved mood, and attention.

Affirming is not about being kind or saying nice things but rather about focusing on some aspect of what the client has done or is doing that you can authentically highlight and affirm. Often what gets affirmed is the process of how the client is behaving, not

https://doi.org/10.1037/0000439-006

Deliberate Practice in Accelerated Experiential Dynamic Psychotherapy, by N. C. N. Prenn, H. Levenson, A. Vaz, and T. Rousmaniere

the content of what is discussed. For example, you could be unequivocally delighted that the client has volunteered how they feel about coming to therapy, even if their feelings are negative. (For example, if the client says, "I really didn't want to come today," you could respond, "I'm so glad you are telling me that.") Sometimes trainees who have learned to be "neutral" or been trained to look for pathology are hesitant about being so openly affirming, delighted, and pleased. It may seem forced or feigned at first; hence, the importance of practicing and seeing how it resonates over time. In AEDP, affirming often includes the self-disclosing of the impact of the client's words on the therapist: "I [the therapist] am delighted."

The therapist's task is to improvise a response to each client statement following these skill criteria:

1. **Match your nonverbal behavior and the quality of your voice (tone, pitch, pacing, rhythm, timbre) with your affirming words.** Matching your voice and body posture to the content of what you are saying is very important in AEDP. Nonlinguistic aspects of the therapist's voice (e.g., its softness) and posture (e.g., leaning in) speak directly to the client's emotional center (Schore, 2019) in a way the words alone cannot. In this communication between the therapist's right hemisphere and the client's right hemisphere, there is a deepening of the client's experience and an undoing their aloneness in the crucible of the relationship. (Also see Exercise 3, "Undoing Aloneness.")

2. **Affirm a specific element of the client's statement.**

SKILL CRITERIA FOR EXERCISE 4

1. Match your nonverbal behavior and prosody (tone) of your voice with your affirming words.
2. Affirm a specific element of the client's statement.

Examples of Therapists Using Affirming

Example 1

CLIENT: [*Proud*] For the first time in a long while, I was able to give myself a break and take a nap instead of overworking.

THERAPIST: [*Smiling broadly*] (Criterion 1) That's so great that you're giving yourself a break! Good for you. (Criterion 2)

Example 2

CLIENT: [*Frustrated*] I'm fed up with how my boss is treating me. I think I really need to address this with her at my next meeting.

THERAPIST: [*Serious and nodding*] (Criterion 1) It's wonderful to hear that you are thinking about being assertive. (Criterion 2)

Example 3

CLIENT: [*Irritated*] I don't see the need to discuss this now.

THERAPIST: [*Nodding*] (Criterion 1) I'm so glad that you can tell me that you don't want to talk about this right now. (Criterion 2)

INSTRUCTIONS FOR EXERCISE 4

Step 1: Role-Play and Feedback

- The client says the first beginner client statement. The therapist **improvises** a response based on the skill criteria.
- The trainer (or, if not available, the client) provides **brief** feedback based on the skill criteria.
- The client then repeats the same statement, and the therapist again improvises a response. The trainer (or client) again provides brief feedback.

Step 2: Repeat

- Repeat Step 1 for all the statements **in the current difficulty level** (beginner, intermediate, or advanced).

Step 3: Assess and Adjust Difficulty

- The therapist completes the Deliberate Practice Reaction Form (see Appendix A) and decides whether to make the exercise easier or harder or to repeat the same difficulty level.

Step 4: Repeat for Approximately 15 Minutes

- Repeat Steps 1 to 3 for at least 15 minutes.
- The trainees then switch therapist and client roles and start over.

> **Now it's your turn! Follow Steps 1 and 2 from the instructions.**

Remember: The goal of the role play is for trainees to practice improvising responses to the client statements in a manner that (a) uses the skill criteria and (b) feels authentic for the trainee. **Example therapist responses for each client statement are provided at the end of this exercise. Trainees should attempt to improvise their own responses before reading the examples.**

BEGINNER CLIENT STATEMENTS FOR EXERCISE 4
Beginner Client Statement 1
[Nodding and smiling] As we talked about last week, I talked to my partner about that thing that has been bothering me. It went really well. Much better than I expected.
Beginner Client Statement 2
[Serious face with a nod] As soon as I found out that I would need to attend the conference, I told my husband that I would be away. He appreciated that I looped him in immediately and didn't avoid telling him.
Beginner Client Statement 3
[Chest heaves, looks sad] I feel so sad about all that I have missed out on in life.
Beginner Client Statement 4
[Proud] I noticed the old self-blaming voice coming up, but I could also feel my anger. It's the first time I realized I'm angry and didn't blame myself.
Beginner Client Statement 5
[Smiling] I felt so proud of myself when she said I had passed. I've wanted to get my driver's license for so long.

> **Assess and adjust the difficulty before moving to the next difficulty level (see Step 3 in the exercise instructions).**

INTERMEDIATE CLIENT STATEMENTS FOR EXERCISE 4
Intermediate Client Statement 1
[Sad] I miss my father so much. It comes up in waves of grief sometimes even all these years later.
Intermediate Client Statement 2
[Angry] I felt humiliated by my mother every single day of my childhood.
Intermediate Client Statement 3
[Irritated] I felt so jealous to hear my friends back home got together without me.
Intermediate Client Statement 4
[Yawn] I can feel myself shutting down as I am talking. It's almost like I'm getting sleepy.
Intermediate Client Statement 5
[Meekly] I can't believe how nervous I was on the stage. My hands were shaking, my voice quavered. I am embarrassed that everyone could tell how scared I was.

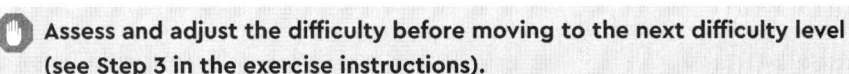 **Assess and adjust the difficulty before moving to the next difficulty level (see Step 3 in the exercise instructions).**

ADVANCED CLIENT STATEMENTS FOR EXERCISE 4
Advanced Client Statement 1
[Nauseous, hand comes up to throat] I really feel like I'm going to throw up. Even thinking about that time makes me want to vomit.
Advanced Client Statement 2
[Broadly smiling] I really felt good after last week's session. I felt so supported and close to you. [Makes eye contact and then quickly looks away] I feel embarrassed saying that.
Advanced Client Statement 3
[Hunched over] Even getting out of bed is hard. Everything feels like a weight right now. [Looks down and hunches over even more] I nearly didn't come to the session today. I just felt like blowing you off.
Advanced Client Statement 4
[Sadly] My mother forgot my birthday again. [Half smiles and bites lip] It's so painful and humiliating. I can't believe how much it still bothers me.
Advanced Client Statement 5
[Leaning forward with serious face] I feel good about being in therapy with you. Things are really changing, and I can't believe I look forward to coming to the sessions. [Big shy smile]

 Assess and adjust the difficulty here (see Step 3 in the exercise instructions). If appropriate, follow the instructions to make the exercise even more challenging (see Appendix A).

Example Therapist Responses: Affirming

Remember: Trainees should attempt to improvise their own responses before reading the examples. **Do not read the following responses verbatim unless you are having trouble coming up with your own!**

EXAMPLE RESPONSES TO BEGINNER CLIENT STATEMENTS FOR EXERCISE 4
Example Response to Beginner Client Statement 1
[Smiling broadly and nodding] (Criterion 1) Wow! This is big! I'm so impressed you talked to your partner, and so glad it went well. Good for you! (Criterion 2)
Example Response to Beginner Client Statement 2
[Smiling and nodding] (Criterion 1) Wow! Good job! We've been working on your telling your husband hard things like that. I am so impressed you did it and glad it went well. (Criterion 2)
Example Response to Beginner Client Statement 3
[Serious face and nodding] (Criterion 1) This is important. You are so full of feeling here. You have missed out. It's brave of you to say so. (Criterion 2)
Example Response to Beginner Client Statement 4
[Smiling and clapping] (Criterion 1) Wow! This is huge. What a big change that you noticed your old protective strategy and also felt the anger. (Criterion 2)
Example Response to Beginner Client Statement 5
[Smiling and thumbs-up sign] (Criterion 1) I am thrilled for you. What an achievement to pass your driving test and get your license. Wow! (Criterion 2)

EXAMPLE RESPONSES TO INTERMEDIATE CLIENT STATEMENTS FOR EXERCISE 4
Example Response to Intermediate Client Statement 1
[Nodding] (Criterion 1) I am so glad you are telling me how much you still miss your father. It's good to talk about this together. (Criterion 2)
Example Response to Intermediate Client Statement 2
[Kind face] (Criterion 1) This is so important. I know it's hard that your mother humiliated you every day, and I am glad we're talking about this. (Criterion 2)
Example Response to Intermediate Client Statement 3
[Gentle nod] (Criterion 1) You are doing such a good job of telling me how you really feel. None of us likes feeling jealous. I appreciate it. (Criterion 2)
Example Response to Intermediate Client Statement 4
[Looking at client intently] (Criterion 1) It is so important that you notice that you're shutting down and getting sleepy. (Criterion 2)
Example Response to Intermediate Client Statement 5
[Slight smile while nodding] (Criterion 1) So brave of you to bring up your stage fright. I appreciate your sharing how nervous you felt. (Criterion 2)

EXAMPLE RESPONSES TO ADVANCED CLIENT STATEMENTS FOR EXERCISE 4
Example Response to Advanced Client Statement 1
[Looking intently] (Criterion 1) This throwing-up feeling is important. You are doing such brave work talking about that time. (Criterion 2)
Example Response to Advanced Client Statement 2
[Slight smile] (Criterion 1) It feels so right to me that you told me how good you felt, and that you felt supported and close to me. (Criterion 2)
Example Response to Advanced Client Statement 3
[Nodding, soft voice] (Criterion 1) I am glad you did come to the session and didn't blow me off. This is a big deal when you feel so weighed down. (Criterion 2)
Example Response to Advanced Client Statement 4
[Nodding seriously] (Criterion 1) You're such a feeling-full person. Of course your mother's forgetting your birthday hurts. (Criterion 2)
Example Response to Advanced Client Statement 5
[Delighted tone] (Criterion 1) You're doing so well and working so hard. Thank you for telling me that being in therapy with me feels good. It's such a big thing that things are really changing. Good for you! (Criterion 2)

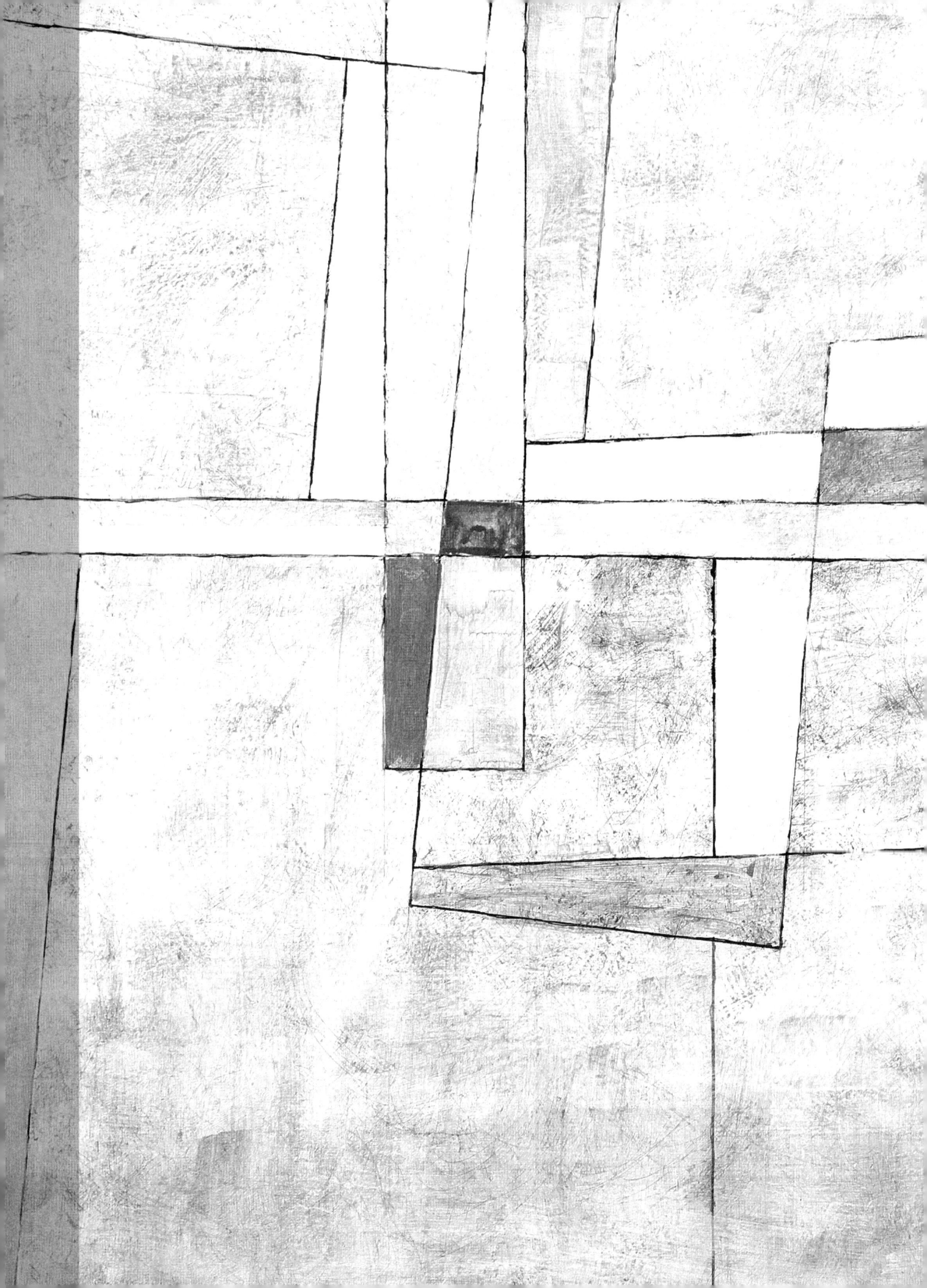

Self-Involving Self-Disclosure

Preparations for Exercise 5

1. Read the instructions in Chapter 2.

2. Download the Deliberate Practice Reaction Form and the Deliberate Practice Diary Form at https://www.apa.org/pubs/books/deliberate-practice-accelerated-experiential-dynamic-psychotherapy (see the "Resources" tab; also available in Appendixes A and B, respectively).

Skill Description

Skill Difficulty Level: Intermediate

Self-disclosure, as a skill, often makes therapists nervous. There is an idea that there is a correct, "neutral" way of working as a psychotherapist, and self-disclosure is breaking that rule. It is important, as we introduce this skill, to define and be clear about what we mean by self-disclosure and how and why we use it in accelerated experiential dynamic psychotherapy (AEDP).

There are two main kinds of self-disclosure. The first, self-involving self-disclosure, happens when the therapist describes their own affect and process, usually in response to something verbal or nonverbal expressed by the client, as it unfolds in the session and from session to session. For example, "When we slow down like this, I feel more connected with you." It is helpful to use a technique that Greenberg and Watson (2006) call "saying all of it" (p. 128). It is not enough to say we feel angry, delighted, or distanced by a client; we need to say all of it and tell the client the specifics, what the content is, and what our process is. We thereby make the implicit explicit and specific. Interventions that demonstrate this idea follow the following format: "When I (see, feel, sense) you do X, then I feel Y."

https://doi.org/10.1037/0000439-007

Deliberate Practice in Accelerated Experiential Dynamic Psychotherapy, by N. C. N. Prenn, H. Levenson, A. Vaz, and T. Rousmaniere

Self-involving self-disclosure accomplishes many AEDP goals. First, it can increase intimacy because the "therapist makes herself vulnerable for the sake of the client and the client's truth" (Russell & Fosha, 2008, p. 181). It can also help create new affective-relational patterns. "It stands to reason that if emotional exchanges, or lack of, create affective patterns that a person creates over and over again, that only new emotional exchanges could facilitate the altering of old affective patterns" (Maroda, 1998, p. 83). Also, emotional exchanges like these allow for the creation of dyadic states of consciousness. "These states of consciousness emerge from the mutual regulation of affect between the client and the therapist. When these dyadic states are achieved, the state of consciousness of the client expands and changes" (Tronick, 1998, p. 298). Self-disclosure is an essential attachment-creating intervention and can be the quickest way to deepen an experience between two people (Prenn, 2009). And finally, therapist self-disclosure shows vulnerability, which can create safety and invite the client to be vulnerable: "disclosure begets disclosure" (Jourard, 1971, p. 16).

As we introduce this skill, it is important to note that it is not the self-disclosure skill alone that can create relationship security; it is the client's response to and experience of the self-disclosure. To learn how a disclosure has landed with a client and to make the self-disclosure therapeutic, we pair this skill with metaprocessing (see Exercise 7), an inquiry and exploration of the impact of the therapist's self-disclosure.

The second type of self-disclosure is called self-revealing. Self-revealing self-disclosure is when a therapist shares their own life experiences, triumphs, vulnerabilities, uncertainties, and dilemmas. Exercise 6 focuses on this second type and will use client statements similar to this exercise so therapists can practice using different types of self-disclosures in the same clinical context.

The therapist's task is to improvise a response to each client statement following these skill criteria:

1. **Be explicit about what the client has said or done to evoke a reaction in you.** In relating how you are feeling, use the standard of "saying all of it"—be sure to include what you are sensing or noticing about the client's nonverbal or verbal behavior. For example, "As you do that, I am feeling this."

2. **Name the reaction/feeling you are having in the moment that is brought on by the client's behavior and/or statements. Use vivid language and be specific.** Such self-disclosing feeling statements may take various forms depending on what is happening with the client. For example, if the client has had an emotional breakthrough and is delighted, you can say how you are moved by the client's joy. On the other hand, when the client is cold and withdrawn, you can say something about how you are feeling held at arm's length. Of course, these statements are said sensitively and with tact to avoid shaming the client.

Remember: Have your nonverbal behavior and tone of your voice consistent with what you are saying. As in the previous exercise, the therapist's use of posture, gesture, facial expression, and qualities of their voice all aid in the client's letting in the therapist's response.

SKILL CRITERIA FOR EXERCISE 5

1. Be explicit about what the client has said or done to evoke a reaction in you.
2. Name the reaction/feeling you are having in the moment that is brought on by the client's behavior and/or statements. Use vivid language and be specific.

Examples of Therapists Using Self-Involving Self-Disclosure

Example 1

CLIENT: [*Joyful*] I feel safer with you now. It feels so good to feel you with me.

THERAPIST: [*Smiling*] I'm so glad to hear it feels good to feel me with you, (Criterion 1) I feel so connected to you. (Criterion 2)

Example 2

CLIENT: [*Touching her heart and looking at the therapist*] I have never told anyone about that horrible experience I had. But I could share it with you because you get it.

THERAPIST: [*Touching their own heart*] When you tell me why you could share that with me, (Criterion 1) I really notice my feelings of warmth for you. (Criterion 2)

Example 3

CLIENT: [*Irritated*] I don't see the need to discuss this now.

THERAPIST: [*Sad*] When you say you don't want to talk about it, (Criterion 1) I feel sad—like I am reaching out to you on one side of a moat and you've pulled up the drawbridge. (Criterion 2)

INSTRUCTIONS FOR EXERCISE 5
Step 1: Role-Play and Feedback
• The client says the first beginner client statement. The therapist **improvises** a response based on the skill criteria.   • The trainer (or, if not available, the client) provides **brief** feedback based on the skill criteria.   • The client then repeats the same statement, and the therapist again improvises a response. The trainer (or client) again provides brief feedback.
Step 2: Repeat
• Repeat Step 1 for all the statements **in the current difficulty** level (beginner, intermediate, or advanced).
Step 3: Assess and Adjust Difficulty
• The therapist completes the Deliberate Practice Reaction Form (see Appendix A) and decides whether to make the exercise easier or harder or to repeat the same difficulty level.
Step 4: Repeat for Approximately 15 Minutes
• Repeat Steps 1 to 3 for at least 15 minutes.   • The trainees then switch therapist and client roles and start over.

Now it's your turn! Follow Steps 1 and 2 from the instructions.

Remember: The goal of the role play is for trainees to practice improvising responses to the client statements in a manner that (a) uses the skill criteria and (b) feels authentic for the trainee. **Example therapist responses for each client statement are provided at the end of this exercise. Trainees should attempt to improvise their own responses before reading the examples.**

BEGINNER CLIENT STATEMENTS FOR EXERCISE 5
Beginner Client Statement 1
[Proudly] I spoke up in class yesterday. A first for me.
Beginner Client Statement 2
[Delighted] I let my partner help me with dinner. It felt good to work on something side by side.
Beginner Client Statement 3
[Satisfied] My kids were frustrating me so much over the weekend, but I kept my cool and didn't yell at them once.
Beginner Client Statement 4
[Proudly] I stayed within budget this month. It helped to keep track of my spending. Thank you for suggesting that app.
Beginner Client Statement 5
[Ashamed] I had a full-on binge on Saturday night. It felt terrible to feel so out of control.

 Assess and adjust the difficulty before moving to the next difficulty level (see Step 3 in the exercise instructions).

INTERMEDIATE CLIENT STATEMENTS FOR EXERCISE 5
Intermediate Client Statement 1
[Sad, shaking head from side to side] I dropped my youngest daughter off at college on Thursday. I thought I'd feel happy and free because we'd been fighting so much, but the house feels kind of empty now. [Big sigh]
Intermediate Client Statement 2
[Frustrated] I feel like I have ADD. I start doing work and the next thing I know I'm on my favorite clothing site looking at shoes.
Intermediate Client Statement 3
[Ashamed, hands over face] I drank too much again last night. I feel like I have a hangover today and feel so ashamed of myself.
Intermediate Client Statement 4
[Angry] My mother phones and just talks about herself. She says she just wants to hear my voice, but it feels more like she wants me to hear *her* voice.
Intermediate Client Statement 5
[Ashamed] I got so mad at my son last night. He has one chore, and he doesn't do it. I feel so bad I yelled at him.

🖐 **Assess and adjust the difficulty before moving to the next difficulty level (see Step 3 in the exercise instructions).**

ADVANCED CLIENT STATEMENTS FOR EXERCISE 5
Advanced Client Statement 1
[Happily, smiling broadly] My mom came for the weekend. We had such a good time. Now that I have learned to set good boundaries with her, I feel much closer to her. It feels so nice!
Advanced Client Statement 2
[Sad, downcast] My best friend gave me the worst gift. How can she not know me? I feel so hurt and confused.
Advanced Client Statement 3
[Angrily] I want to be perfect. I can't stand that I am afraid of flying. It's irrational and honestly makes me feel weak.
Advanced Client Statement 4
[Shoulders rounded, sad] There is always a depressed place in me. Like even when I am happy I can touch into the center of me and it's sad and down in there. I don't think it'll ever change.
Advanced Client Statement 5
[Frustrated] I was on the phone with my electric company for 5 hours yesterday. I wasted the whole day. I could cry. I'm so angry.

> **Assess and adjust the difficulty here (see Step 3 in the exercise instructions). If appropriate, follow the instructions to make the exercise even more challenging (see Appendix A).**

Example Therapist Responses: Self-Involving Self-Disclosure

Remember: Trainees should attempt to improvise their own responses before reading the examples. **Do not read the following responses verbatim unless you are having trouble coming up with your own!**

EXAMPLE RESPONSES TO BEGINNER CLIENT STATEMENTS FOR EXERCISE 5
Example Response to Beginner Client Statement 1
As you talk about your courageous act of speaking up, (Criterion 1) I feel like cheering. (Criterion 2)
Example Response to Beginner Client Statement 2
When you tell me about how good it felt to work side by side with your partner, (Criterion 1) I found myself smiling broadly. (Criterion 2)
Example Response to Beginner Client Statement 3
I can feel your victory in my heart. (Criterion 2) What an accomplishment to keep your cool in the face of their uproar. (Criterion 1)
Example Response to Beginner Client Statement 4
Hearing how you used my suggestion in such a fruitful manner (Criterion 1) makes me feel we are working beautifully together. (Criterion 2)
Example Response to Beginner Client Statement 5
Listening to how you felt out of control with your drinking (Criterion 1) at first made me hold my breath. And then I could feel myself breathing again, realizing that you were inviting me into what it was like for you. (Criterion 2)

EXAMPLE RESPONSES TO INTERMEDIATE CLIENT STATEMENTS FOR EXERCISE 5

Example Response to Intermediate Client Statement 1

As you tell me how you are really feeling versus what you were anticipating feeling, (Criterion 1) I realize how far you have come in allowing yourself to be present with whatever is going on inside you. (Criterion 2)

Example Response to Intermediate Client Statement 2

Your describing to me what you notice about your behavior (Criterion 1) really makes me feel like I have a partner in this work we are doing together. (Criterion 2)

Example Response to Intermediate Client Statement 3

I feel how ashamed you are. (Criterion 1) It sounds funny to say, but I am glad you are sharing this with me. (Criterion 2)

Example Response to Intermediate Client Statement 4

Oh ow! I feel angry at her too. (Criterion 1) I appreciate you for telling me exactly where we need to be. (Criterion 2)

Example Response to Intermediate Client Statement 5

I feel how bad you feel. (Criterion 1) I feel pained on your behalf. (Criterion 2)

EXAMPLE RESPONSES TO ADVANCED CLIENT STATEMENTS FOR EXERCISE 5
Example Response to Advanced Client Statement 1
It feels so nice inside of me (Criterion 2) to hear how close you feel to your mom as a result of our work together. (Criterion 1)
Example Response to Advanced Client Statement 2
Your hurt is palpable. (Criterion 1) I feel so pained on your behalf. (Criterion 2)
Example Response to Advanced Client Statement 3
When you tell me how you feel, (Criterion 1) I feel like we are teamed up together. (Criterion 2)
Example Response to Advanced Client Statement 4
I feel so close to you (Criterion 2) when you tell me what your experience is. (Criterion 1)
Example Response to Advanced Client Statement 5
I know how frustrating that is. (Criterion 2) I am so glad you are telling me. (Criterion 1)

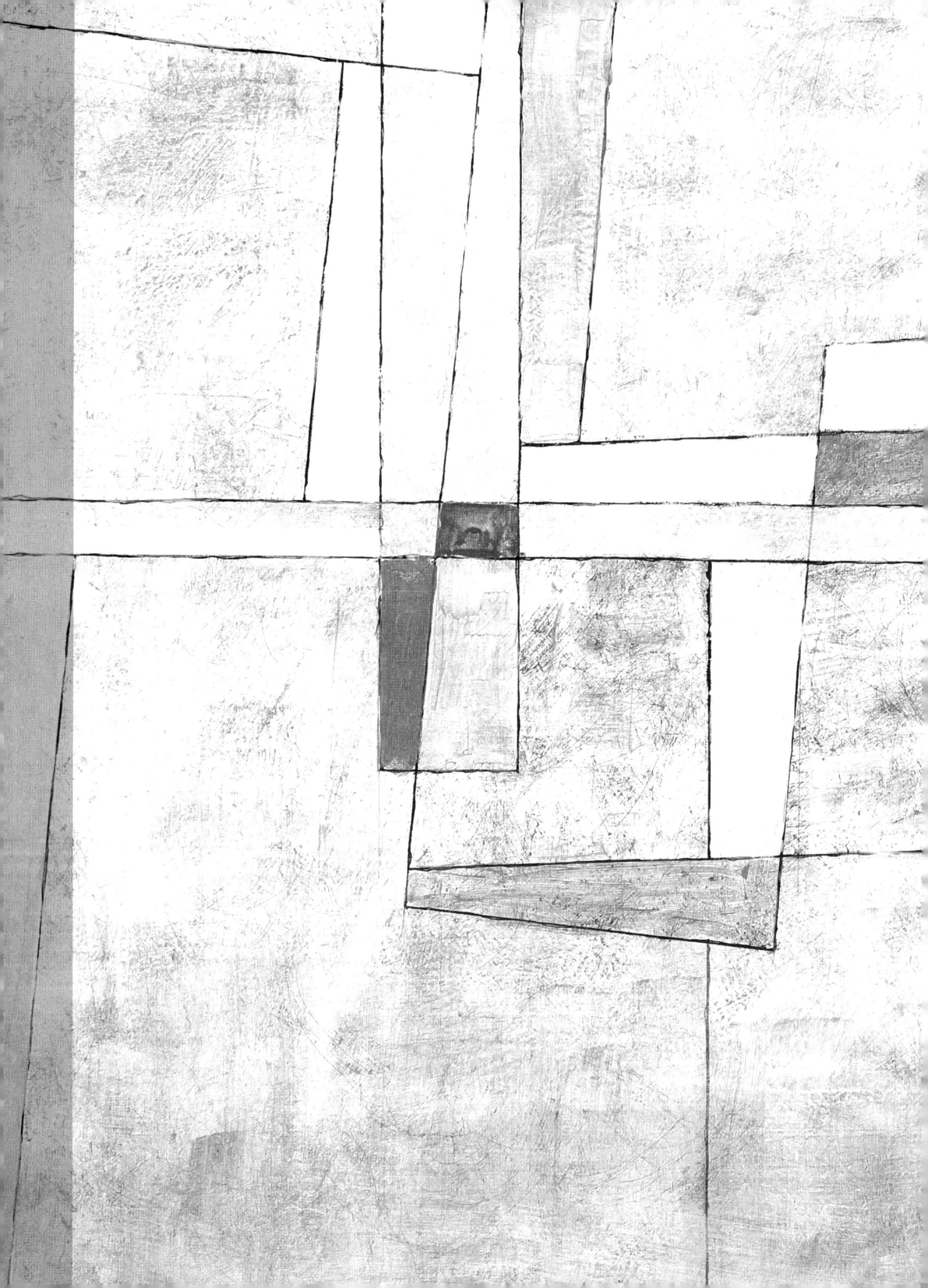

Self-Revealing Self-Disclosure

Preparations for Exercise 6

1. Read the instructions in Chapter 2.

2. Download the Deliberate Practice Reaction Form and the Deliberate Practice Diary Form at https://www.apa.org/pubs/books/deliberate-practice-accelerated-experiential-dynamic-psychotherapy (see the "Resources" tab; also available in Appendixes A and B, respectively).

Skill Description

Skill Difficulty Level: Intermediate

Exercise 5, "Self-Involving Self-Disclosure," speaks to how the therapist is affected by what the client is saying. This exercise's skill focuses on another type of self-disclosure. *Self-revealing self-disclosure* is when the therapist shares something personal about their own experience that relates to the essence of what the client is saying. It is a way of saying, "I know what this is like. The two of us have this in common." Research (Hill & Knox, 2001; Knox et al., 1997) has indicated that this type of self-disclosure can have a powerful impact on client insight, make the therapist "seem more real and human," and lead to more client openness. From an accelerated experiential dynamic psychotherapy (AEDP) point of view, self-revealing self-disclosures can be a building block to deepening the relationship and contain the essence of an empathic response. "I, too, have walked in your shoes."

Self-revealing self-disclosures are powerful interventions, and so it is important to emphasize that we use them sparingly and judiciously and always in the service of the client. There are many more times in an actual therapy session when you wouldn't self-disclose at all or would keep the self-disclosure very general, especially around "hot topics," like sex and violence. For more guidance, see the Helpful Hints box.

---

https://doi.org/10.1037/0000439-008

Deliberate Practice in Accelerated Experiential Dynamic Psychotherapy, by N. C. N. Prenn, H. Levenson, A. Vaz, and T. Rousmaniere

In AEDP, whenever possible, we pair self-disclosure with metaprocessing—asking the client about how hearing this personal information from the therapist impacted them. You will get to practice metaprocessing in Exercise 7. For now, let's focus on this skill of self-revealing self-disclosure.

The therapist's task is to improvise a response to each client statement following this skill criterion:

1. **Share your own personal experience that relates to the most poignant or significant part of the client's statement.** For this skill the therapist mentions their actual life experiences, triumphs, vulnerabilities, uncertainties, and dilemmas that relate to what the client is expressing (see the Helpful Hints box).

SKILL CRITERION FOR EXERCISE 6

Share your own personal experience that relates to the most poignant or significant part of the client's statement.

HELPFUL HINTS

1. Some of the client statements in this exercise are the same as those in Exercise 5, but here you will get to try a personal rather than an interpersonal intervention.

2. Although this exercise focuses solely on using self-revealing self-disclosures, we recommend that in your actual therapy sessions, you use them sparingly, and when you do, that you do not overshare—in particular, avoid being explicit about very personal experiences (e.g., sexual behaviors).

3. As usual in AEDP, match the energy of the client's statement. Let the client cue your tone, pitch, and pacing.

Examples of Therapists Using Self-Revealing Self-Disclosures

Example 1

CLIENT: [*Calmly*] I feel safer with you now. It feels so good to feel you with me.

THERAPIST: I know from my own experience how good it feels to feel safe with my therapist.

Example 2

CLIENT: [*Ashamed*] I felt so jealous hearing that my friends back home got together without me.

THERAPIST: Oh, that is hard; I have felt that kind of jealousy too.

Example 3

CLIENT: [*Sad*] I miss my father so much. It comes up in waves of grief sometimes even all these years later.

THERAPIST: I know how that feels. I have lost a parent. Grief still comes up for me sometimes.

INSTRUCTIONS FOR EXERCISE 6

Step 1: Role-Play and Feedback

- The client says the first beginner client statement. The therapist **improvises** a response based on the skill criterion.
- The trainee (or, if not available, the client) provides **brief** feedback based on the skill criterion.
- The client then repeats the same statement, and the therapist again improvises a response. The trainee (or client) again provides brief feedback.

Step 2: Repeat

- Repeat Step 1 for all the statements **in the current difficulty level** (beginner, intermediate, or advanced).

Step 3: Assess and Adjust Difficulty

- The therapist completes the Deliberate Practice Reaction Form (see Appendix A) and decides whether to make the exercise easier or harder or to repeat the same difficulty level.

Step 4: Repeat for Approximately 15 Minutes

- Repeat Steps 1 to 3 for at least 15 minutes.
- The trainees then switch therapist and client roles and start over.

> ➡️ **Now it's your turn! Follow Steps 1 and 2 from the instructions.**

Remember: The goal of the role play is for trainees to practice improvising responses to the client statements in a manner that (a) uses the skill criteria and (b) feels authentic for the trainee. **Example therapist responses for each client statement are provided at the end of this exercise. Trainees should attempt to improvise their own responses before reading the examples.**

BEGINNER CLIENT STATEMENTS FOR EXERCISE 6
Beginner Client Statement 1
[Proudly] I spoke up in class yesterday. A first for me.
Beginner Client Statement 2
[Delighted] I let my partner help me with dinner. It felt good to work on something side by side.
Beginner Client Statement 3
[Satisfied] My kids were frustrating me so much over the weekend, but I kept my cool and didn't yell at them once.
Beginner Client Statement 4
[Proudly] I stayed within budget this month. It helped to keep track of my spending. Thank you for suggesting that app.
Beginner Client Statement 5
[Ashamed] I had a full-on binge on Saturday night. It felt terrible to feel so out of control.

> ✋ **Assess and adjust the difficulty before moving to the next difficulty level (see Step 3 in the exercise instructions).**

INTERMEDIATE CLIENT STATEMENTS FOR EXERCISE 6
Intermediate Client Statement 1
[Sadly shaking head from side to side] I dropped my youngest daughter off at college on Thursday. I thought I'd feel happy and free because we'd been fighting so much, but the house feels kind of empty now. [Big sigh]
Intermediate Client Statement 2
[Frustrated] I feel like I have ADD: I start doing work and the next thing I know I'm on my favorite clothing site looking at shoes.
Intermediate Client Statement 3
[Ashamed, hands over face] I drank too much again last night. I feel like I have a hangover today and feel so ashamed of myself.
Intermediate Client Statement 4
[Angry] My mother phones and just talks about herself. She says she just wants to hear my voice, but it feels like she just wants me to hear her voice.
Intermediate Client Statement 5
[Ashamed] I got so mad at my son last night. He has one chore, and he doesn't do it. I feel so bad I yelled at him.

 Assess and adjust the difficulty before moving to the next difficulty level (see Step 3 in the exercise instructions).

ADVANCED CLIENT STATEMENTS FOR EXERCISE 6
Advanced Client Statement 1
[Smiling broadly] I had the best sex of my life last night!
Advanced Client Statement 2
[Sad, downcast] My best friend gave me the worst gift. How can she not know me? I feel so hurt and confused.
Advanced Client Statement 3
[Angrily] I want to be perfect. I can't stand that I am afraid of flying. It's irrational and honestly makes me feel weak.
Advanced Client Statement 4
[Shoulders rounded, sad] There is always a depressed place in me. Like even when I am happy, I can touch into the center of me, and it's sad and down in there. I don't think I can really keep feeling this way much longer.[1]
Advanced Client Statement 5
[Angry] I am so angry at my ex-wife, I feel like I could punch her.

 Assess and adjust the difficulty here (see Step 3 in the exercise instructions). If appropriate, follow the instructions to make the exercise even more challenging (see Appendix A).

---

1. Expressions such as "I don't think I can really keep feeling this way much longer" may reflect a feeling and not an intent to harm oneself. Nevertheless, therapists need to use a multitude of contextual client indicators to determine suicidal intent. Trainees should seek close supervision for clients who may be at risk for self-harm or suicide.

Example Therapist Responses: Self-Revealing Self-Disclosures

Remember: Trainees should attempt to improvise their own responses before reading the examples. **Do not read the following responses verbatim unless you are having trouble coming up with your own!**

EXAMPLE RESPONSES TO BEGINNER CLIENT STATEMENTS FOR EXERCISE 6
Example Response to Beginner Client Statement 1
That's great! Good for you. I have struggled with speaking up in class, so I know what a big deal that is.
Example Response to Beginner Client Statement 2
You let your partner help. From one control freak to another, [smile] I know how hard it is to let someone help and how good sharing an activity like cooking can feel!
Example Response to Beginner Client Statement 3
That is a big achievement. I know how frustrating little kids can be and how good it feels when I can keep my cool.
Example Response to Beginner Client Statement 4
You stayed within your budget! Great! I love that app too. It has really helped me.
Example Response to Beginner Client Statement 5
Argh. Feeling out of control feels so bad. I know what that feels like too.

EXAMPLE RESPONSES TO INTERMEDIATE CLIENT STATEMENTS FOR EXERCISE 6
Example Response to Intermediate Client Statement 1
Oh, wow! I remember having a very similar feeling when I dropped off my youngest too.
Example Response to Intermediate Client Statement 2
Oh, that happens to me sometimes. I try to ask myself what was going on before I found myself shopping! I wonder what was going on for you.
Example Response to Intermediate Client Statement 3
Ack. I'm with you. I've been to therapy feeling out of it. How is it for you?
Example Response to Intermediate Client Statement 4
When someone calls and just talks about themselves it makes me feel angry too.
Example Response to Intermediate Client Statement 5
Teenagers are the worst! I have lost my cool with my own kids. It feels terrible.

EXAMPLE RESPONSES TO ADVANCED CLIENT STATEMENTS FOR EXERCISE 6
Example Response to Advanced Client Statement 1
That is great! I know how enjoyable it is to have a wonderful romantic experience. (**Reminder:** Keep self-disclosure about sex vague and general rather than matching specific content.)
Example Response to Advanced Client Statement 2
I'm so happy for you! I know what you mean. A gift can really make you feel seen. I love that feeling.
Example Response to Advanced Client Statement 3
Wanting perfection. I know that one too. Our stuff is a bit different. I know what it's like dealing with a big fear.
Example Response to Advanced Client Statement 4
That is a hard place to be. I've had experiences of really being sad as well. And let's be thorough and discuss what you said about not being sure you can really keep feeling this way much longer. [Use self-disclosure and then explore potential for self-harm/suicide]
Example Response to Advanced Client Statement 5
Wow, I know what it's like to feel really angry at someone. (**Reminder:** Keep self-disclosure general and at an emotional level rather than refer to specific acts of physical violence.)

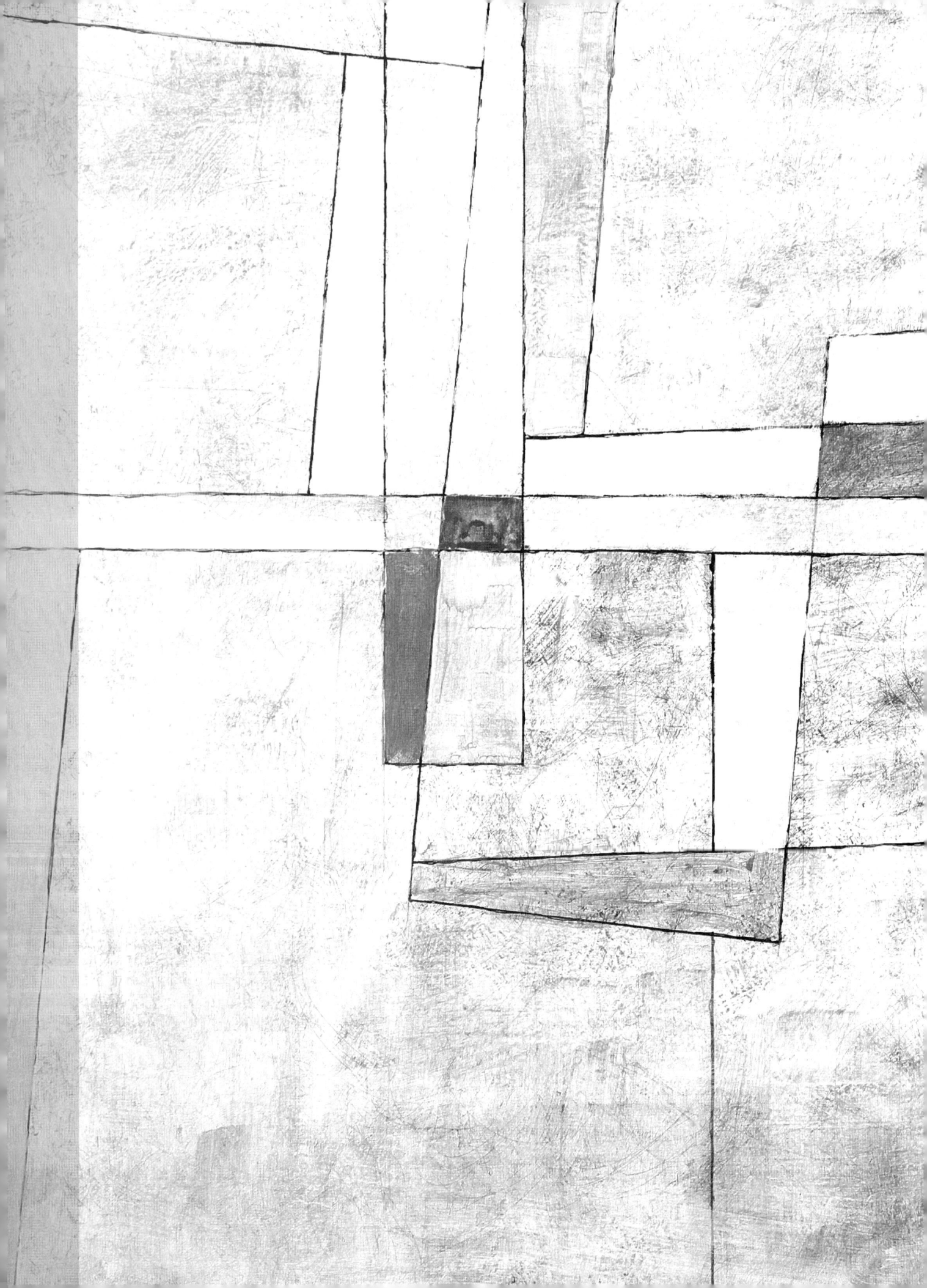

Metaprocessing

Preparations for Exercise 7

1. Read the instructions in Chapter 2.

2. Download the Deliberate Practice Reaction Form and the Deliberate Practice Diary Form at https://www.apa.org/pubs/books/deliberate-practice-accelerated-experiential-dynamic-psychotherapy (see the "Resources" tab; also available in Appendixes A and B, respectively).

Skill Description

Skill Difficulty Level: Intermediate

Metaprocessing is used to focus in on a very specific moment that is happening between therapist and client, and inquire about it, without trying to figure it out or having preconceived ideas about what it might mean. This is a skill we use frequently in accelerated experiential dynamic psychotherapy (AEDP). Think of it as an "add-on" to almost any skill to check out how the client is experiencing what is happening in the therapy. This skill usually involves a question that is designed to check in systematically about the therapy process as the therapy unfolds.

The standard metaprocessing question inquires about the effect of a therapist's behavior on the client. "So what is this like for you right now that I noticed X [or said Y or did Z]?" The reverse, asking about the client's experience of their own behavior, can also be metaprocessed. "What's it like for you that you did X [or said Y] in here with me just now?" When the client answers, it starts a central process of further inquiry. Metaprocessing is the second intervention in almost everything we do in AEDP because what is critical is how the client experiences what is happening moment-to-moment in the therapy. Depending on what the client says, the therapist will know what interventions need to happen next (e.g., further processing, repair of a rupture, undoing aloneness, affirmation).

https://doi.org/10.1037/0000439-009

Deliberate Practice in Accelerated Experiential Dynamic Psychotherapy, by N. C. N. Prenn, H. Levenson, A. Vaz, and T. Rousmaniere

In this way, metaprocessing makes implicit interactions explicit. It helps clients know that we can look at, inquire into, and talk about the experiences that are happening between therapist and client, self to self, and everything in between. The goal is to set in motion corrective emotional and relational interactions.

In this exercise, we focus on exploring interactions between the therapist and client, especially the client's response to an intervention made by the therapist: "What's that like for you inside that I noticed your holding your breath?" "What's it like that I asked you to stay with your sadness just now?" "What is it like for you that I am being challenging about this right now?" The exploration can also focus on a particularly "juicy" (affect-laden) word voiced by the client or a nonverbal movement, gesture, or other reaction, including a lack of movement or reaction (e.g., a sigh, a flushing of the face, an immobile facial expression).

Metaprocessing brings the client's relational dynamics into the therapy to facilitate "portable change" for clients outside therapy. Additionally, if a client's responses to metaprocessing indicate a rupture in the therapy relationship (e.g., "I felt self-conscious when you noticed I looked away while talking"), it can be processed and repaired, which fosters a healthy process and positive outcomes.

In AEDP, there are two ways of examining client–therapist interactions in the moment. The first is what we are covering in this exercise, *metaprocessing*, which is a way of examining and then fine-tuning moment-to-moment interactions on a microlevel. The second type is *metatherapeutic processing*, which is used when the client has had experiences of positive therapeutic change and the work focuses on the emergent positive emotion that arises from that experience in session. We introduce the skill of metatherapeutic processing in Exercise 12. In the AEDP literature, "metaprocessing" is sometimes used as if it were shorthand for "metatherapeutic processing" (e.g., Fosha, 2021, p. 5; Iwakabe et al., 2020, p. 550). But we wish to make this distinction because they are fundamentally two different skills. (See also Prenn, 2011, p. 310.)

The therapist's task is to improvise a response to each client statement following these skill criteria:

1. **Make an intervention.** For this skill practice, because metaprocessing is what the AEDP therapist does next, we are going to use client statements similar to those you have already in previous exercises so that you can make an intervention (i.e., moment-to-moment tracking, affirming, or self-disclosure), and then use metaprocessing to inquire about how that intervention landed. We have divided the client statements into three categories: the five beginner statements ask you to track moment-to-moment (Skill 1) and then metaprocess; the five intermediate statements ask you to affirm (Skill 4) and then metaprocess; and the five advanced statements ask you to use self-revealing self-disclosure (Skill 6) and then metaprocess.

2. **Ask the client to reflect on their internal experience of the therapist's intervention.** Here the therapist asks the client to focus on their experience (thoughts, feelings, somatic sensations) just after the therapist has done or said something in the here-and-now of the session. The therapist maintains a stance of curiosity in making the inquiry.

SKILL CRITERIA FOR EXERCISE 7

1. Make an intervention:
   - **Option A:** Moment-to moment tracking
   - **Option B:** Affirming
   - **Option C:** Self-revealing self-disclosure
2. Ask the client to reflect on their internal experience of the therapist's intervention.

Examples of Therapists Using Metaprocessing

Example 1: Moment-to-Moment Tracking

CLIENT: [*Shy, biting their thumb nail*] I really like being in therapy with you.

THERAPIST: You start biting your thumb nail as you say that. (Criterion 1, Option A) What's it like for you that I notice that? (Criterion 2)

Example 2: Affirming

CLIENT: [*Proud*] For the first time in a long while, I was able to give myself a break and take a nap instead of overworking.

THERAPIST: That's so great that you're giving yourself a break! I'm so delighted. Good for you. (Criterion 1, Option B) What's it like for you that I said, "Good for you?" (Criterion 2)

Example 3: Self-Revealing Self-Disclosure

CLIENT: [*Irritated*] I don't see the need to discuss this now.

THERAPIST: When I hear you say you don't want to talk about it, I feel sad—like I'm reaching out to you on one side of a moat and you've pulled up the drawbridge. (Criterion 1, Option C) How is it to hear the impact your words are having on me? (Criterion 2)

INSTRUCTIONS FOR EXERCISE 7

Step 1: Role-Play and Feedback

- The client says the first beginner client statement. The therapist **improvises** a response based on the skill criteria.

- The trainee (or, if not available, the client) provides **brief** feedback based on the skill criteria.

- The client then repeats the same statement, and the therapist improvises a response. The trainee (or client) again provides brief feedback.

Step 2: Repeat

- Repeat Step 1 for all the statements **in the current difficulty level** (beginner, intermediate, or advanced).

Step 3: Assess and Adjust Difficulty

- The therapist completes the Deliberate Practice Reaction Form (see Appendix A) and decides whether to make the exercise easier or harder or to repeat the same difficulty level.

Step 4: Repeat for Approximately 15 Minutes

- Repeat Steps 1 to 3 for at least 15 minutes.
- The trainees then switch therapist and client roles and start over.

> **Now it's your turn! Follow Steps 1 and 2 from the instructions.**

Remember: The goal of the role play is for trainees to practice improvising responses to the client statements in a manner that (a) uses the skill criteria and (b) feels authentic for the trainee. **Example therapist responses for each client statement are provided at the end of this exercise. Trainees should attempt to improvise their own responses before reading the examples.**

Note: In these five beginner statements, ask trainees to track, moment-to-moment, and then metaprocess.

BEGINNER CLIENT STATEMENTS FOR EXERCISE 7
Beginner Client Statement 1
[Meek, rounding their shoulder and hunching] It was a better week, [pause] I think.
Beginner Client Statement 2
It was a great vacation! **[Big sigh]** We had a very good time together.
Beginner Client Statement 3
[Big breath in to keep from crying] I miss him so much.
Beginner Client Statement 4
[Placing a hand over their heart] An image of my childhood home keeps coming to my mind; it was such a calm and happy place.
Beginner Client Statement 5
[Making fists with both hands] She just leaves the dishes in the sink. I am so sick of her self-centered ways. Does she just expect me to clean up after her?

> **Assess and adjust the difficulty before moving to the next difficulty level (see Step 3 in the exercise instructions).**

Note: In these five intermediate statements, ask trainees to affirm then metaprocess.

INTERMEDIATE CLIENT STATEMENTS FOR EXERCISE 7
Intermediate Client Statement 1
[Exasperated] I hate it when you ask me how I feel inside. I've told you. I don't feel anything! Stop asking me!
Intermediate Client Statement 2
[Angry] I am so pissed off at you right now. I feel like you're saying I should break up with my boyfriend, and I really don't think it's your place to tell me what to do.
Intermediate Client Statement 3
[Serious, looking at therapist] I really felt good after last week's session. I felt so supported and close to you. **[Looks away]** I feel embarrassed saying that.
Intermediate Client Statement 4
[Proud] I noticed the old self-blaming voice coming up, but I could also feel my anger. It's the first time I realized I'm angry and didn't blame myself.
Intermediate Client Statement 5
[Sad] My mother forgot my birthday again. **[Half smiles and bites lip]** It's so painful, and humiliating. And I can't believe how much it still bothers me.

🖐 **Assess and adjust the difficulty before moving to the next difficulty level (see Step 3 in the exercise instructions).**

Note: In these five advanced statements, ask trainees to self-disclose then metaprocess.

ADVANCED CLIENT STATEMENTS FOR EXERCISE 7
Advanced Client Statement 1
[Ashamed] I felt so jealous to hear my friends back home got together without me.
Advanced Client Statement 2
[Sad] I miss my father so much. It comes up in waves of grief sometimes even all these years later.
Advanced Client Statement 3
[Frustrated] I was on the phone with my electric company for 5 hours yesterday. I wasted the whole day. I could cry. I'm so angry.
Advanced Client Statement 4
[Happy, smiling broadly] My mom came for the weekend. We had such a good time. Now that I have learned to set good boundaries with her, I feel much closer to her. It feels so nice.
Advanced Client Statement 5
[Sad] I feel so sad at how my girlfriend treats me.

 Assess and adjust the difficulty here (see Step 3 in the exercise instructions). If appropriate, follow the instructions to make the exercise even more challenging (see Appendix A).

Example Therapist Responses: Metaprocessing

Remember: Trainees should attempt to improvise their own responses before reading the examples. **Do not read the following responses verbatim unless you are having trouble coming up with your own!**

EXAMPLE RESPONSES TO BEGINNER CLIENT STATEMENTS FOR EXERCISE 7 MOMENT-TO-MOMENT TRACKING FOLLOWED BY METAPROCESSING
Example Response to Beginner Client Statement 1
You round your shoulders and hunch right over as you say that. (Criterion 1, Option A) What's it like that I notice that? (Criterion 2)
Example Response to Beginner Client Statement 2
That's a big sigh . . . (Criterion 1, Option A) What's it like that I noticed your sigh? (Criterion 2)
Example Response to Beginner Client Statement 3
You hold your breath and hold back your tears. (Criterion 1, Option A) What's it like that I notice that? (Criterion 2)
Example Response to Beginner Client Statement 4
You put a hand over your heart. (Criterion 1, Option A) How is it for you that I notice that? (Criterion 2)
Example Response to Beginner Client Statement 5
You're making fists with your hands. (Criterion 1, Option A) How does it feel inside that I notice that? (Criterion 2)

EXAMPLE RESPONSES TO INTERMEDIATE CLIENT STATEMENTS FOR EXERCISE 7 AFFIRMING FOLLOWED BY METAPROCESSING
Example Response to Intermediate Client Statement 1
Thank you for telling me. It is so helpful when you're direct like this. (Criterion 1, Option B) How is it to know that your directness helps me and our work together? (Criterion 2)
Example Response to Intermediate Client Statement 2
I really appreciate your telling me this. (Criterion 1, Option B) How is it to know I welcome your directness? (Criterion 2)
Example Response to Intermediate Client Statement 3
You are so brave in telling me when you feel embarrassed to say it. (Criterion 1, Option B) How is it to hear how brave I think you are? (Criterion 2)
Example Response to Intermediate Client Statement 4
Wow! This is huge. What a big change that you noticed your old protective strategy and also felt the anger. (Criterion 1, Option B) How is it that I am sharing in your pride? (Criterion 2)
Example Response to Intermediate Client Statement 5
You are such a feelingful person in all the best ways. Of course it bothers you. She's your mother! (Criterion 1, Option B) How is it for you that I say that? (Criterion 2)

EXAMPLE RESPONSES TO ADVANCED CLIENT STATEMENTS FOR EXERCISE 7
SELF-REVEALING SELF-DISCLOSURE FOLLOWED BY METAPROCESSING

Example Response to Advanced Client Statement 1

Oh, that is hard; I have felt that kind of jealousy too. (Criterion 1, Option C) What is that like for you to know that I have felt jealous like that too? (Criterion 2)

Example Response to Advanced Client Statement 2

I know how that feels. I have lost a parent. Grief still comes up for me in waves sometimes. (Criterion 1, Option C) What's it like to know that about me? (Criterion 2)

Example Response to Advanced Client Statement 3

I have had that experience too. Hours on the phone. I know how frustrating that is. (Criterion 1, Option C) What is it like to know I've been there too? (Criterion 2)

Example Response to Advanced Client Statement 4

I feel full of smiles inside of me to hear how close you feel to your mom as a result of our work together. (Criterion 1, Option C) What does it feel like for you that I feel full of smiles? (Criterion 2)

Example Response to Advanced Client Statement 5

Hearing that, I feel sad in my heart too. (Criterion 1, Option C) What is it like to hear I feel sad for you? (Criterion 2)

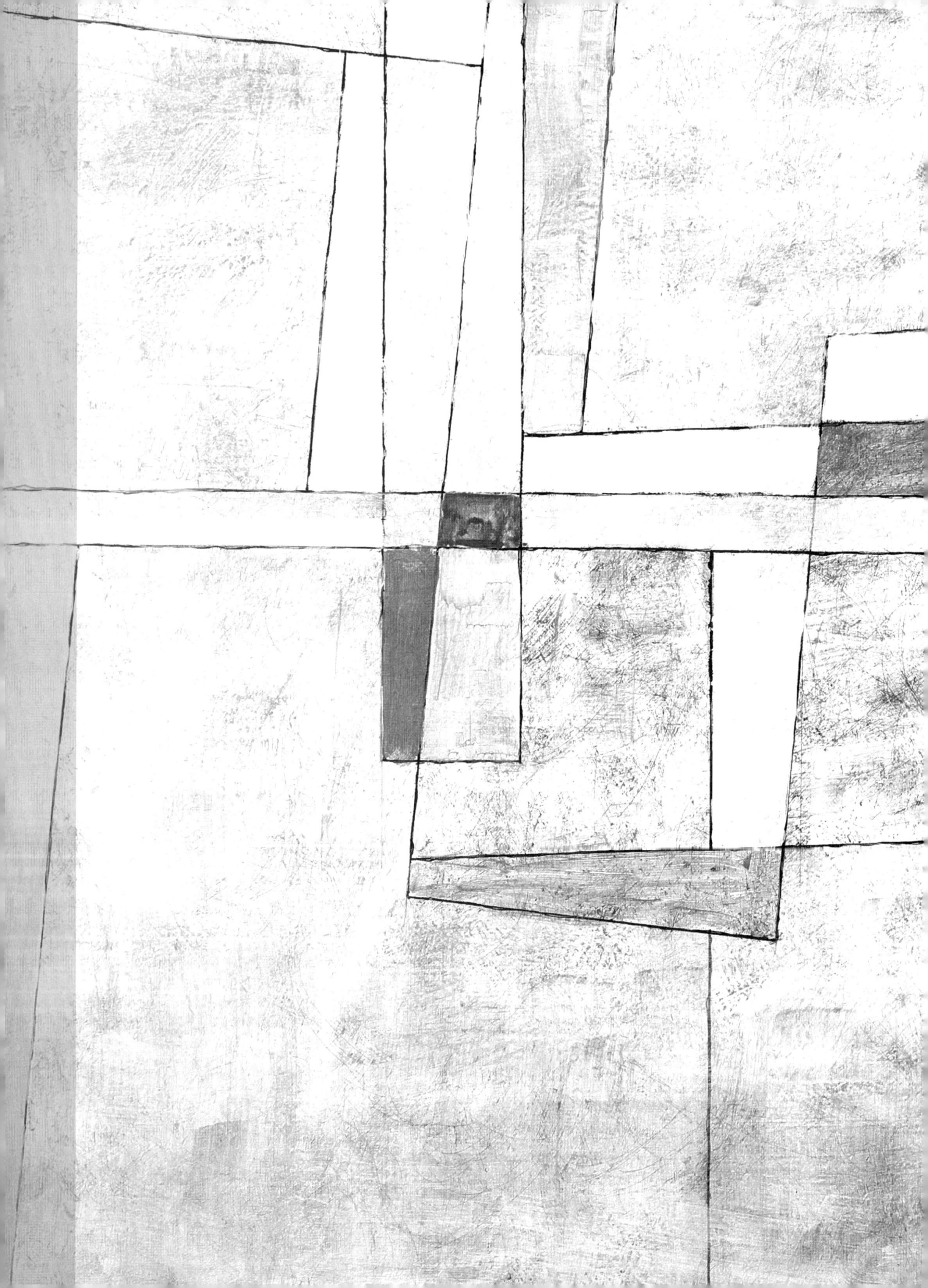

Working With Anxiety

Preparations for Exercise 8

1. Read the instructions in Chapter 2.

2. Download the Deliberate Practice Reaction Form and the Deliberate Practice Diary Form at https://www.apa.org/pubs/books/deliberate-practice-accelerated-experiential-dynamic-psychotherapy (see the "Resources" tab; also available in Appendixes A and B, respectively).

Skill Description

Skill Difficulty Level: Advanced

Working with anxiety is a central skill in accelerated experiential dynamic psychotherapy (AEDP). As we try to help clients feel their internal visceral experience of themselves, they will probably start to feel anxious. In AEDP, we want to keep our foot on the gas pedal of anxiety. Some therapists may wonder, "But why? Isn't anxiety bad? Isn't our function as therapists to lessen it?" Not necessarily. Anxiety tells us something important is coming up and we want to find a way to (re)educate clients that, from the perspective of emotion theory, anxiety can be an informative place for understanding when and why we are avoiding certain activities, thoughts, and feelings.

We would like to help patients experience anxiety as a healthy signal from their bodies and not something to be feared, suppressed, or medicated away. When I (N. P.) was first learning AEDP, as clients became anxious, I would work too quickly to regulate their anxiety. I was afraid, if they became uncomfortable, that somehow I was doing something wrong or something that might hurt them. All my clients were regulated, but over time I realized that this was working to keep them distant from their core feelings.

https://doi.org/10.1037/0000439-010

Deliberate Practice in Accelerated Experiential Dynamic Psychotherapy, by N. C. N. Prenn, H. Levenson, A. Vaz, and T. Rousmaniere

I learned that anxiety comes up as the client–therapist dyad moves into emotional territory, and I now know this is an important place to be. Now I reframe anxiety as often essential for the therapeutic work. Eileen Russell (2021) concurs:

> Many patients actually need to learn to tolerate their anxiety without resorting to defenses to allow themselves to have new experiences both intrapsychically and interpersonally. As long as we are within the window of tolerance, it is okay to push, encourage, and proceed, instead of feeling the need to back off. *People can be too regulated to grow.* (p. 258, emphasis added)

There is an exception to this stance of inviting and using anxiety as it manifests in the work. If the client is clearly overwhelmed, then you do want to downregulate their anxiety. In this case, many of the skills in this book will help lessen anxiety by supporting the client's self-righting capacities in the context of dyadic regulation (e.g., undoing aloneness, self-disclosing, affirming).

This exercise focuses on how to make use of anxiety in two circumstances. The first circumstance is when the client is aware of the anxiety and lets the therapist know, for example "I'm feeling pretty anxious right now." The second circumstance is when the patient is not consciously aware that they are anxious, but the anxiety becomes apparent through the client's body or voice (e.g., leg jiggling, stammering, fast talking).

The therapist's task is to improvise a response to each client statement following these skill criteria:

1. **Reframe the anxiety, however it manifests, as positive.** Psychoeducation that anxiety holds important information is useful to clients and helps them notice it, get to know it, tolerate it, and learn from it. Examples of explaining anxiety's purpose include "Anxiety lets us know something important is coming up," "It may sound counterintuitive, but anxiety is your body signaling that we are in the right place," and "Anxiety is helping us know this is important."

2. **Ask permission to explore.** After explaining that anxiety is an important physical experience to pay attention to, ask the client if it is alright with them to explore it. Examples include "Would it be okay with you if we paid attention to the anxiety and got to know it?" "Can we explore the anxiety?" and "What's it like physically?"

SKILL CRITERIA FOR EXERCISE 8

1. Reframe the anxiety, however it manifests, as positive.
2. Ask permission to explore the anxiety.

Examples of Therapists Working With Anxiety

Example 1

CLIENT: [*Nervous*] I am feeling pretty anxious right now. [pause] You know, I didn't have any breakfast this morning. Maybe if I get some food in me, I will feel better.

THERAPIST: Your anxiety is a good sign that something important is coming up. (Criterion 1) Can we listen to what the anxiety is about? (Criterion 2)

Example 2

CLIENT: [*Biting fingernails*] I'm feeling so thirsty—like my throat is totally dry.

THERAPIST: Hmm. Sounds like your body might be alerting us that something important is coming up right now. (Criterion 1) I'm wondering if it would be okay with you if we tune into the messages from your body? (Criterion 2)

Example 3

CLIENT: I feel so jittery. I think I'd best take a chill pill right now.

THERAPIST: I'm wondering before you reach for a pill, if you could focus on that jittery feeling for just a moment? (Criterion 2) Sometimes those jittery feelings contain such good information for us. (Criterion 1)

INSTRUCTIONS FOR EXERCISE 8

Step 1: Role-Play and Feedback

- The client says the first beginner client statement. The therapist **improvises** a response based on the skill criteria.
- The trainee (or, if not available, the client) provides **brief** feedback based on the skill criteria.
- The client then repeats the same statement, and the therapist again improvises a response. The trainee (or client) again provides brief feedback.

Step 2: Repeat

- Repeat Step 1 for all the example statements **in the current difficulty level** (beginner, intermediate, or advanced).

Step 3: Assess and Adjust Difficulty

- The therapist completes the Deliberate Practice Reaction Form (see Appendix A) and decides whether to make the exercise easier or harder or to repeat the same difficulty level.

Step 4: Repeat for Approximately 15 Minutes

- Repeat Steps 1 to 3 for at least 15 minutes.
- The trainees then switch therapist and client roles and start over.

Now it's your turn! Follow Steps 1 and 2 from the instructions.

Remember: The goal of the role play is for trainees to practice improvising responses to the client statements in a manner that (a) uses the skill criteria and (b) feels authentic for the trainee. **Example therapist responses for each client statement are provided at the end of this exercise. Trainees should attempt to improvise their own responses before reading the examples.**

BEGINNER CLIENT STATEMENTS FOR EXERCISE 8
Beginner Client Statement 1
[Nervous] I am feeling pretty anxious right now. [pause] You know, I didn't have any breakfast this morning. Maybe if I get some food in me, I will feel better.
Beginner Client Statement 2
[Massaging neck] I've just been feeling so tense all day.
Beginner Client Statement 3
[Puzzled] I don't know why, but I've just been on edge all day.
Beginner Client Statement 4
[Anxious] I think I'm kind of nervous today. It just started in the waiting room.
Beginner Client Statement 5
[Curious] Something is definitely going on with me right now. All of a sudden, I got really worried, but I don't know about what.

Assess and adjust the difficulty before moving to the next difficulty level (see Step 3 in the exercise instructions).

INTERMEDIATE CLIENT STATEMENTS FOR EXERCISE 8
Intermediate Client Statement 1
[Curious] All of a sudden, I'm feeling so thirsty—like my throat is totally dry.
Intermediate Client Statement 2
[Fingers repeatedly tapping on both legs] How are you today?
Intermediate Client Statement 3
[Talking rapidly] So I just saw the most amazing sunset on my way over here and it was just so beautiful and I almost missed the bus but I made it, and I am so happy to be here, and I don't know what to talk about and . . .
Intermediate Client Statement 4
[Hesitating speech] Hmm. [pause] Do you think? [pause] I mean, what do you think about? [pause] Ah, I forgot what I was going to say.
Intermediate Client Statement 5
[Fanning themself with a hand] All of sudden I feel kind of flushed. Is it hot in here? I need to take off my jacket.

 Assess and adjust the difficulty before moving to the next difficulty level (see Step 3 in the exercise instructions).

ADVANCED CLIENT STATEMENTS FOR EXERCISE 8
Advanced Client Statement 1
[Shaky hands] I feel so jittery. I think I'm going to take a chill pill.
Advanced Client Statement 2
[Worried] You know I can hear my heart beating. It feels like my heart is just going to pop out of my chest like in a cartoon version of myself.
Advanced Client Statement 3
[Curious] I woke up this morning with this enormous sense of dread. I can't remember ever having it before. It's scaring me. Is it a premonition of something awful?
Advanced Client Statement 4
[Anxious] I'm feeling kind of lightheaded right now and a bit dizzy.
Advanced Client Statement 5
[Panicky] I am having this series of thoughts in my mind right now that you are not well and might be dying. I never thought that before! Are you okay?

> **Assess and adjust the difficulty here (see Step 3 in the exercise instructions). If appropriate, follow the instructions to make the exercise even more challenging (see Appendix A).**

Example Therapist Responses: Working With Anxiety

Remember: Trainees should attempt to improvise their own responses before reading the examples. **Do not read the following responses verbatim unless you are having trouble coming up with your own!**

EXAMPLE RESPONSES TO BEGINNER CLIENT STATEMENTS FOR EXERCISE 8
Beginner Client Statement 1
Your anxiety is a good sign that something important is coming up. (Criterion 1) Can we listen to what the anxiety is about? (Criterion 2)
Beginner Client Statement 2
Could we listen to your muscles right now to hear what they might be saying? (Criterion 2) Because sometimes the tension in our bodies carries important information for us about what we are feeling. (Criterion 1)
Beginner Client Statement 3
Hmm. I don't know why either. But it sounds important. (Criterion 1) Could we take some time to focus on what it is like for you being on edge all day? (Criterion 2)
Beginner Client Statement 4
Great that you know what is going on inside and when it began. (Criterion 1) Would it be okay with you to describe that nervousness that just began in the waiting room? (Criterion 2)
Beginner Client Statement 5
That's important. (Criterion 1) Could we spend a couple of minutes exploring that worried feeling? (Criterion 2)

EXAMPLE RESPONSES TO INTERMEDIATE CLIENT STATEMENTS FOR EXERCISE 8
Intermediate Client Statement 1
Hmm. Sounds like your body might be alerting us that something important is coming up right now. (Criterion 1) I'm wondering if it would be okay with you if we tune into the messages from your dry throat. (Criterion 2)
Intermediate Client Statement 2
I'm wondering if your tapping fingers want to say something right now that could be helpful? (Criterion 1) Could we take a listen? (Criterion 2)
Intermediate Client Statement 3
It sounds pretty amazing alright, but I'm also noticing how rapidly you are talking and wonder if we could pay attention to that? (Criterion 2) Sometimes how we say things is as important as exactly what we are saying. (Criterion 1)
Intermediate Client Statement 4
So something is really wanting to interrupt your talking right now. (Criterion 1) Do you think you could leave some room for the pauses and see what comes up? (Criterion 2)
Intermediate Client Statement 5
Hmm. Maybe there is something your body wants to let you know right now—sort of like highlighting. (Criterion 1) What comes to mind, if you just let it? (Criterion 2)

EXAMPLE RESPONSES TO ADVANCED CLIENT STATEMENTS FOR EXERCISE 8

Advanced Client Statement 1

I'm wondering before you take the pill, if you could focus on that jittery feeling for just a moment. (Criterion 2) Sometimes those jittery feelings contain such good information for us. (Criterion 1)

Advanced Client Statement 2

It sounds like your heart really wants to be heard right now. It's beating so loudly. (Criterion 1) Could we tune into your heart and see if it's trying to tell us something important? (Criterion 2)

Advanced Client Statement 3

Before we try to figure out if it is a negative thing, what about exploring it (Criterion 2) to see what value it might have for our work? (Criterion 1)

Advanced Client Statement 4

I'm right here. Could the two of us together explore this dizzy feeling? (Criterion 2) I have a sense that it has some wisdom for us. (Criterion 1)

Advanced Client Statement 5

Yes, I am fine, but you are having these thoughts for some reason. (Criterion 1) Could you talk about these thoughts and see what we can make of them? (Criterion 2)

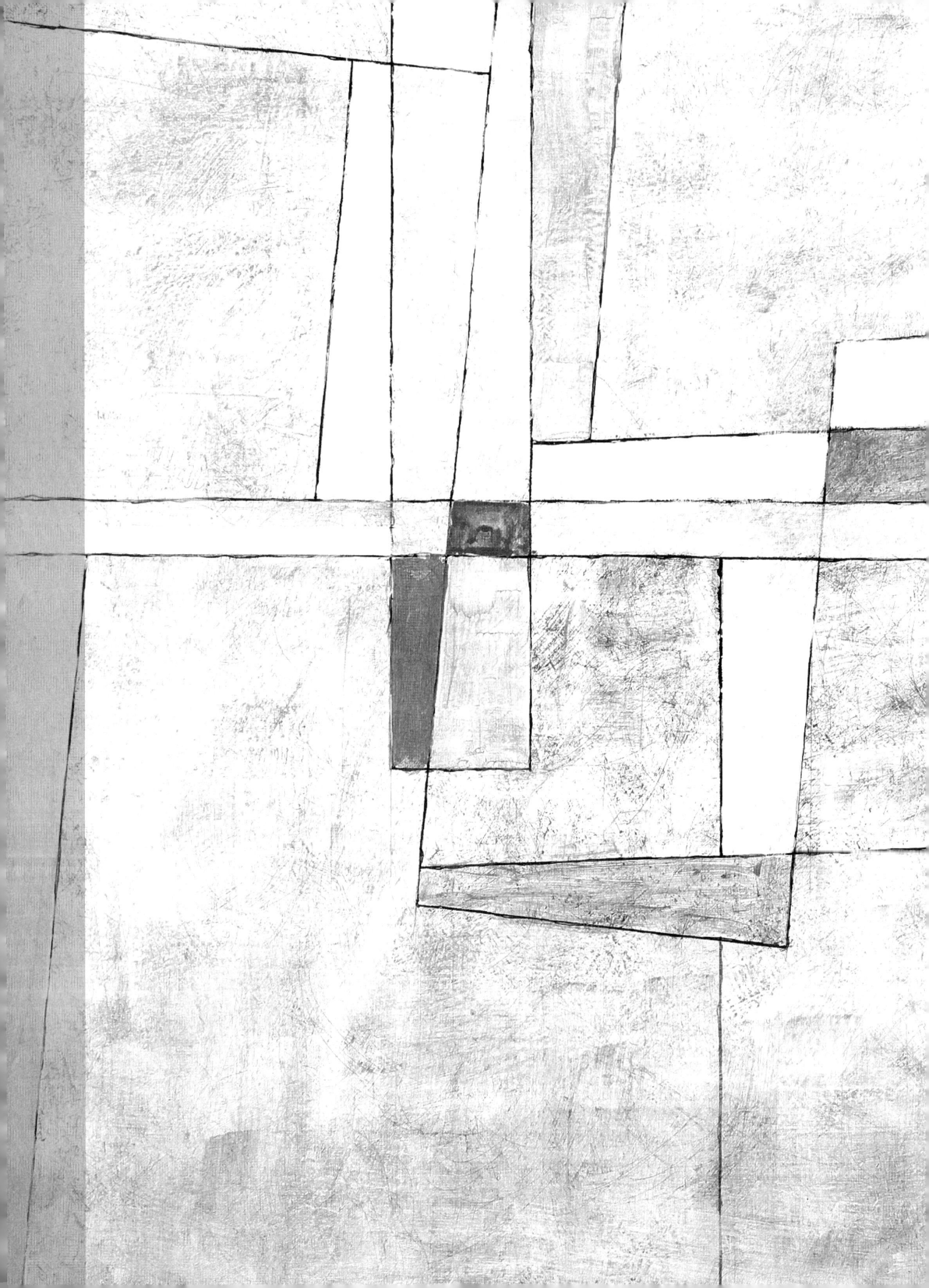

Affirmative Work With Defenses

Preparations for Exercise 9

1. Read the instructions in Chapter 2.

2. Download the Deliberate Practice Reaction Form and the Deliberate Practice Diary Form at https://www.apa.org/pubs/books/deliberate-practice-accelerated-experiential-dynamic-psychotherapy (see the "Resources" tab; also available in Appendixes A and B, respectively).

Skill Description

Skill Difficulty Level: Advanced

Many clients present in therapy relying on defensive strategies that helped them at one phase of their lives but now are not working or are overworking, which causes symptoms and problems. One way to help shift defenses is by using the transforming power of experiencing core feelings and relational affects. Explicitly being with the client (the skill of undoing aloneness from Exercise 3) is one way that accelerated experiential dynamic psychotherapy (AEDP) therapists bypass and melt defenses.

In affirmatively working with defenses, therapists explicitly appreciate and celebrate the client's defenses. In AEDP we do not go to war with defenses; we try hard not to shame clients for strategies that were probably brilliantly adaptive for them growing up but now are getting in their way. In addition to validating a developmental need for a defense, the AEDP therapist helps the client be curious about the defense and helps them focus on staying with the primary affect and connecting with the therapist rather than defending against feeling and relational closeness.

https://doi.org/10.1037/0000439-011

Deliberate Practice in Accelerated Experiential Dynamic Psychotherapy, by N. C. N. Prenn, H. Levenson, A. Vaz, and T. Rousmaniere

The therapist's task is to improvise a response to each client statement using the following skill criteria:

1. **Describe what the client does instead of feeling the primary affect.** Notice how the defense comes up in the session. Describing what the client does in a nonevaluative manner often invites the client to be curious about the use of the defense. For example, "You are saying you are so angry and yet you smile" or "When I ask you how you feel about your father, your mind goes blank."

2. **Value the defense in the client's present or past.** The AEDP therapist views defenses as self-protective acts, usually learned in childhood. Therapists value the defense by celebrating it—affirming ("loving up") its need, validating it, or expressing gratitude to it.

3. **Invitation to action.**

    • **Option A:** Invite the client to explore the defense. For example, "If that [defensive] part of you could speak to us right now, what would it want to say?" or "What does your wall feel like?"

    • **Option B:** Invite the client to bypass the defense. For example, "If for just a moment, we put that [the defense] to the side, what else do you notice?" "What else comes up?" "What else do you feel?" "Would that part of you be willing to step aside for just a moment?" or "Can we see what happens if we put that aside for just a moment?"

SKILL CRITERIA FOR EXERCISE 9

1. Describe what the client does instead of feeling the primary affect.
2. Value the defense in the client's present or past.
3. Invitation to action:

    • **Option A:** Invite the client to explore the defense.
    • **Option B:** Invite the client to bypass the defense.

HELPFUL HINT

If for Criterion 3 you see yourself (or if your role-play partner sees you) favoring one option over another, you might challenge yourself by trying the less-used option.

Examples of Affirmative Work With Defenses

Example 1

CLIENT: [*Confused*] When you ask me how I feel about my father, my mind goes blank.

THERAPIST: So when I ask you how you feel about your father, your mind goes blank. (Criterion 1) How brilliant that your mind could do that for you! (Criterion 2) And if that blanking out part of your mind could speak to us right now, what does it say? (Criterion 3, Option A)

or

If we put the blankness to the side, what comes up? (Criterion 3, Option B)

Example 2

CLIENT: [*Smiling*] I always feel the same. I'm miserable.

THERAPIST: You say you're miserable and you smile. (Criterion 1) Wow, there must be a good reason for you to smile. (Criterion 2) How does it feel to smile when you're so miserable? (Criterion 3, Option A)

or

And if you didn't smile, what is the miserableness like? (Criterion 3, Option B)

Example 3

CLIENT: [*Angry*] I'm so mad at my roommate. She keeps using all my stuff. She used all my soap last month and I had to buy more, and now she's using the new soap I bought! She's so annoying. I mean. I don't know. But you know what I mean. [Shrug and smile]

THERAPIST: Sounds like you are mad at her! And then you shrug and say you don't know. (Criterion 1) My guess is that shrugging and getting vague was a useful strategy growing up. (Criterion 2) Right now, here with me, how is it to shrug and get vague and say I don't know? (Criterion 3, Option A)

or

What if we stayed with being mad at her, and don't shrug and get vague? (Criterion 3, Option B)

INSTRUCTIONS FOR EXERCISE 9

Step 1: Role-Play and Feedback

- The client says the first beginner client statement. The therapist **improvises** a response based on the skill criteria.
- The trainee (or, if not available, the client) provides **brief** feedback based on the skill criteria.
- The client then repeats the same statement, and the therapist improvises a response. The trainee (or client) again provides brief feedback.

Step 2: Repeat

- Repeat Step 1 for all the statements **in the current difficulty level** (beginner, intermediate, or advanced).

Step 3: Assess and Adjust Difficulty

- The therapist completes the Deliberate Practice Reaction Form (see Appendix A) and decides whether to make the exercise easier or harder or to repeat the same difficulty level.

Step 4: Repeat for Approximately 15 Minutes

- Repeat Steps 1 to 3 for at least 15 minutes.
- The trainees then switch therapist and client roles and start over.

Now it's your turn! Follow Steps 1 and 2 from the instructions.

Remember: The goal of the role play is for trainees to practice improvising responses to the client statements in a manner that (a) uses the skill criteria and (b) feels authentic for the trainee. **Example therapist responses for each client statement are provided at the end of this exercise. Trainees should attempt to improvise their own responses before reading the examples.**

BEGINNER CLIENT STATEMENTS FOR EXERCISE 9
Beginner Client Statement 1
[Clenched jaw with anger] I'm so angry I feel sort of frozen, like I can't move—like it's created an immobility in me.
Beginner Client Statement 2
[Big smile and direct eye contact] I felt so good after our last session. I felt like you really understood me. I felt close to you. [Looks down and covers their face with both hands]
Beginner Client Statement 3
[Angry] I'd like to punch him. I really would. He makes me so mad. [Apologetic] I mean I don't want to punch him. I'm not a violent person.
Beginner Client Statement 4
[Thoughtful] I felt really proud after the meeting. They seemed to really like my ideas. I was humming and singing as I was walking down the street afterward. And then that negative voice came in saying, "This won't last. They didn't like you that much. Don't get carried away."
Beginner Client Statement 5
[Matter of fact] I guess I should be feeling sad right now. The breakup is so recent, but I try to brush it off. So many things in my life are positive too, you know. Other people have suffered much worse than a breakup, you know.

 Assess and adjust the difficulty before moving to the next difficulty level (see Step 3 in the exercise instructions).

INTERMEDIATE CLIENT STATEMENTS FOR EXERCISE 9
Intermediate Client Statement 1
[Earnest] I'm feeling pretty good. And yet, I can feel myself keeping a lid on the good feeling like it's dangerous to let myself feel too good. [Laughs and covers face]
Intermediate Client Statement 2
[Angry] They never drive to see me. So I have to drive an hour each way to see them. I mean, it's fine. It really is. Don't get me wrong, I love to drive.
Intermediate Client Statement 3
[Disgusted] When you say you don't know what advice to give me, I feel like you're weak and I feel kind of disgusted with you. It's difficult to acknowledge even to myself how disgusted I feel. I know I am overreacting and it's irrational.
Intermediate Client Statement 4
[Tentative] I was on cloud nine. I was so happy and then that feeling came up of unease, anxiety, like I wasn't safe.
Intermediate Client Statement 5
[Angry, shaking a fist] She's taking me to the cleaners financially. I can't stand her. She's the reason we're getting divorced, and she's still getting the apartment and all this money. [Looks sad, sighs deeply, shoulders slump] But giving her the money is what I have to do.

 Assess and adjust the difficulty before moving to the next difficulty level (see Step 3 in the exercise instructions).

ADVANCED CLIENT STATEMENTS FOR EXERCISE 9

Advanced Client Statement 1

[**Complaining**] No one ever helps me. I have to do everything by myself and I'm good at it, so it works, but I'm so tired. The trouble is, none of my colleagues can really do any of the stuff I can do, so I have to do it all myself.

Advanced Client Statement 2

[**Angry**] I hate when you ask me how I feel about things in that therapist-y, compassionate way. I know you think I should be sad. You're trying to get me to cry. It makes me angry.

Advanced Client Statement 3

[**Arms across chest, shoulders rounded**] I'm so angry. My ex texted me last night criticizing me about my parenting. I couldn't sleep at all after I read it. [pause] You know, throughout this session my stomach has been gnawing at me. I feel so hungry. Is there somewhere close by I could get something to eat?

Advanced Client Statement 4

[**Suspicious**] I got really uncomfortable about how you greeted me in the waiting room. You seemed so glad to see me. I'm sure you're being phony.

Advanced Client Statement 5

[**Matter-of-fact**] My doctor sent me here. He thinks I'm pretty depressed and drinking too much. But actually, I'm quite happy with my life. I have a few drinks. Too many drinks sometimes for sure, but my life is good. I'm happy.

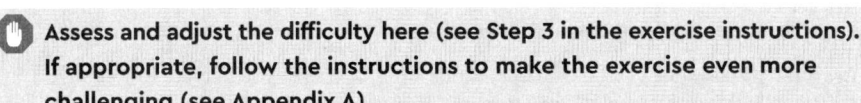 **Assess and adjust the difficulty here (see Step 3 in the exercise instructions). If appropriate, follow the instructions to make the exercise even more challenging (see Appendix A).**

Example Therapist Responses: Affirmative Work With Defenses

Remember: Trainees should attempt to improvise their own responses before reading the examples. **Do not read the following responses verbatim unless you are having trouble coming up with your own!**

EXAMPLE RESPONSES TO BEGINNER CLIENT STATEMENTS FOR EXERCISE 9
Example Response to Beginner Client Statement 1
You get frozen. (Criterion 1) I'm sure there's a good reason you've done that. (Criterion 2) What's the frozen feeling like? (Criterion 3, Option A) or And if you let yourself defrost, and feel the anger, what's it like? (Criterion 3, Option B)
Example Response to Beginner Client Statement 2
I am so glad you felt good and close to me, and like I really understand you. And something's happening right now as you tell me—you smile and then you look down and you cover your face with your hands. (Criterion 1) I'm sure there's a good reason you look down and cover your face. (Criterion 2) What's happening inside as you look down and cover your face? (Criterion 3, Option A) or If you stay with me and the big smile, what's it like? (Criterion 3, Option B)
Example Response to Beginner Client Statement 3
You feel mad and then you take it back. (Criterion 1) Of course you're mad. (Criterion 2) What happens inside when you feel mad and then take it back? (Criterion 3, Option A) or What if you didn't take it back and we stayed with the punch? (Criterion 3, Option B)
Example Response to Beginner Client Statement 4
You feel proud and then something happens inside. (Criterion 1) Such a protective voice comes up. I'm sure it kept you safe growing up. (Criterion 2) Walk me into that moment when you felt proud and the negative voice came up. What was it like? (Criterion 3, Option A) or Can we stay with the proud? (Criterion 3, Option B)
Example Response to Beginner Client Statement 5
You guess you should be feeling sad right now and yet you try to focus on the positive and compare your pain with other people's. (Criterion 1) This was such a good way to not feel sad growing up. (Criterion 2) What's it like to try to brush it off and focus on the positive? (Criterion 3, Option A) or If you didn't try to brush it off, what's the sadness like? (Criterion 3, Option B)

EXAMPLE RESPONSES TO INTERMEDIATE CLIENT STATEMENTS FOR EXERCISE 9

Example Response to Intermediate Client Statement 1

You're feeling pretty good and yet you put on a lid to keep yourself from feeling too good. (Criterion 1) I can understand why it feels dangerous to let yourself feel too good given your early years. (Criterion 2) What is the lid like? Can we get to know it together? (Criterion 3, Option A)

or

If you took the lid off in here with me right how, what's the good feeling like? (Criterion 3, Option B)

Example Response to Intermediate Client Statement 2

So you focus on your love of driving, and you say it's fine. (Criterion 1) Given your experiences growing up, I can understand your not counting on others to do their share. (Criterion 2) So can you tell me about your love of driving and how you don't mind doing it all the time? (Criterion 3, Option A)

or

If you didn't feel like driving one day, I wonder what you might be feeling about their not coming to see you. (Criterion 3, Option B)

Example Response to Intermediate Client Statement 3

You feel disgusted at me, and it's hard to acknowledge it even to yourself, and then you dismiss your true feeling by saying you're overreacting or irrational. (Criterion 1) Criticizing your feelings and calling yourself irrational was a good strategy because when you were young, voicing your true feelings would have rocked the boat at home. (Criterion 2) What happens when you just let yourself feel the disgust and don't criticize yourself for it? (Criterion 3, Option A)

or

And now here with me can we do it differently by acknowledging to yourself that you think I'm weak and it brings up disgust in you? (Criterion 3, Option B)

Example Response to Intermediate Client Statement 4

You were on cloud nine and then that feeling came up. (Criterion 1) Given how happiness was so fleeting growing up, you brilliantly protected yourself from feeling it for very long. (Criterion 2) Can we get to know the anxiety? (Criterion 3, Option A)

or

And what if we stay with the cloud nine feeling, the happy feeling and ask the anxiety not to come in? (Criterion 3, Option B)

Example Response to Intermediate Client Statement 5

You say you can't stand her, then you kind of collapse. (Criterion 1) It's safer not being angry; a lesson you learned growing up. (Criterion 2) What if we interviewed the part of you that collapses? (Criterion 3, Option A)

or

And now here with me, can we do it differently? If you sat up straight, and I'll do it too, to see what happens. (Criterion 3, Option B)

EXAMPLE RESPONSES TO ADVANCED CLIENT STATEMENTS FOR EXERCISE 9

Example Response to Advanced Client Statement 1

[Soft voice] You have to do everything by yourself because no one else is up to the task. (Criterion 1) Your self-reliance has served you so well throughout your life. (Criterion 2) What does the "I have to do it myself" feel like inside? (Criterion 3, Option A)

or

And if your colleagues come forward and could really help you, what is that like? (Criterion 3, Option B)

Example Response to Advanced Client Statement 2

[Soft voice] So when I ask you about your feelings in a therapist-y way, it makes you angry. (Criterion 1) I can understand why you would get angry thinking I want to make you cry. (Criterion 2) What is it like to be upset with me? (Criterion 3, Option A)

or

And if we could momentarily ignore the therapist-y way I asked you the question, I'm wondering if you could go back to how you felt when I asked you how you were feeling about something possibly so sad? (Criterion 3, Option B)

Example Response to Advanced Client Statement 3

So your ex texted and criticized you. And you couldn't sleep thinking about it. Now you tell me you feel hungry. (Criterion 1) My guess is that you were feeling something when you couldn't sleep, but instead of talking about that feeling here, you focus on your body, much like you did when you were kid when it wasn't safe to talk about feelings. (Criterion 2) Can we get to know what the gnawing feels like? (Criterion 3, Option A)

or

And if you didn't focus on the hunger and let whatever you were feeling when you couldn't sleep come up, what would that be like? (Criterion 3, Option B)

Example Response to Advanced Client Statement 4

My greeting you warmly felt uncomfortable to you. (Criterion 1) I am sure you come by this discomfort and then suspicion honestly. (Criterion 2) Can you tell me more about the uncomfortableness? (Criterion 3, Option A)

or

What if I really were that glad to see you? (Criterion 3, Option B)

Example Response to Advanced Client Statement 5

You want to make sure I know that you are not depressed but happy. (Criterion 1) Focusing on how happy you are sounds like it has kept you quite positive throughout your life. (Criterion 2) What does it feel like to feel happy and have a few too many drinks? (Criterion 3, Option A)

or

Maybe right now, if you don't worry about classifying yourself as happy or sad, could you just tell me about you? (Criterion 3, Option B)

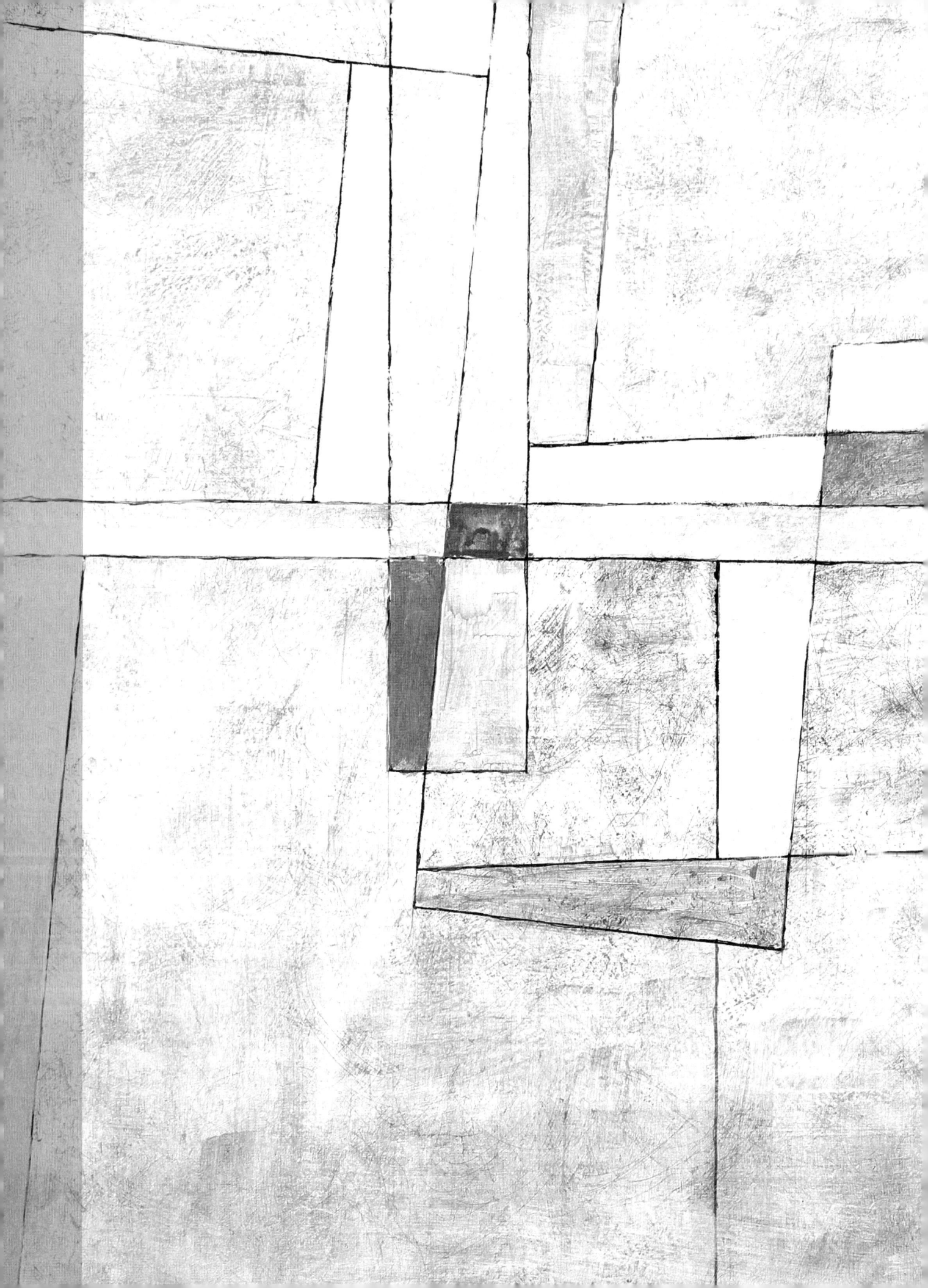

Initiating Portrayals

Preparations for Exercise 10

1. Read the instructions in Chapter 2.

2. Download the Deliberate Practice Reaction Form and the Deliberate Practice Diary Form at https://www.apa.org/pubs/books/deliberate-practice-accelerated-experiential-dynamic-psychotherapy (see the "Resources" tab; also available in Appendixes A and B, respectively).

Skill Description

Skill Difficulty Level: Advanced

In accelerated experiential dynamic psychotherapy (AEDP), we use portrayals as a technique to process emotions and to access unconscious dynamic material. A portrayal is a role-play technique that sets up a monologue or interaction either interpersonally through addressing an imagined person (real or fictitious) or with a part of the self intrapsychically. The more vivid and specific the imagery of the portrayal through the five senses, the more the client can connect affectively to what they are experiencing (Pally & Olds, 2000). Portrayals are used to rework or complete "unfinished business" with another or with the self (Greenberg & Malcolm, 2002) or work an unprocessed emotion such as anger and grief to completion. Portrayals are not meant for a client to rehearse something to say to someone in the client's life although over time, they do help clients expand their capacities to be assertive or express more vulnerable feelings. To clarify this to clients, therapists can say, "This is an exercise to help you get in touch with your feelings. It is not a rehearsal for action in real life. This is for us here together to know how you really feel. Over time, it is intended to help you expand your capacities to feel and express yourself."

https://doi.org/10.1037/0000439-012

Deliberate Practice in Accelerated Experiential Dynamic Psychotherapy, by N. C. N. Prenn, H. Levenson, A. Vaz, and T. Rousmaniere

The therapist's task is to improvise a response to each client statement following these skill criteria:

1. **Invite the client to imagine a person or part of the self, bringing in details of that person or part.** Invite the client to experience that person or part of the self in some sensory and/or visceral detail. Make sure that the client is immersed in the experience of addressing the person or part of the self. Helping the client make the image vivid (e.g., what the "person" is wearing, how they sound, what scent they are wearing) and promoting the visceral quality of the interaction (e.g., the queasiness in the pit of the stomach) will help the portrayal come alive and often foster a cascade of emotion.

2. **Invite the client to address this imagined person or part directly.** Say something simple, such as "So what would you want to say to X if you just let yourself?" If you think the client might have trouble getting started, you can suggest some beginning words, such as "Tell your father, 'Dad, I am really angry with you,'" or "Let that part of you sitting there on the couch know, 'I really want you to pay attention to what I am about to say.'"

SKILL CRITERIA FOR EXERCISE 10

1. Invite the client to imagine a person or part of the self, bringing in details of that person or part.
2. Invite the client to address this imagined person or part directly.

HELPFUL HINTS

1. It can help build the reality of the setting for the dialogue if you gesture toward a chair where the imagined person (part of the self) can sit and direct the client to look and talk directly toward the imagined person (part) sitting there.
2. Similarly, it can also make the portrayal more real if the therapist is also looking at the imagined person or back and forth from the imagined person to the client, rather than just at the client.

Examples of Therapists Setting Up Portrayals

Example 1

CLIENT: [*Angry*] The holiday weekend was terrible—we all fought. My father was particularly enraging, [shakes a fist in the air] and we spent the whole weekend walking on eggshells around him.

THERAPIST: So if you imagined your father right here with us right now, (Criterion 1) what does your fist want to do to him and what would you say to him? (Criterion 2)

Example 2

CLIENT: [*Looking down, regretful*] My boss always picks on me. She is so mean. I always shut down around her and can't speak up.

THERAPIST: So if we imagine her here right now, I want you to visualize what she is wearing and how she is standing. (Criterion 1) What would you speak up and say to her? (Criterion 2**)**

Example 3

CLIENT: [*Sadly*] I was such a lonely kid. Particularly in second grade when my brother had so many emotional problems.

THERAPIST: So if you imagined that second grader—really imagined that young child with their hair and clothes—looking so lonely, (Criterion 1) what would you say or do to help that child feel less lonely? (Criterion 2)

INSTRUCTIONS FOR EXERCISE 10

Step 1: Role-Play and Feedback

- The client says the first beginner client statement. The therapist **improvises** a response based on the skill criteria.
- The trainer (or, if not available, the client) provides **brief** feedback based on the skill criteria.
- The client then repeats the same statement, and the therapist again improvises a response. The trainer (or client) again provides brief feedback.

Step 2: Repeat

- Repeat Step 1 for all the example statements **in the current difficulty level** (beginner, intermediate, or advanced).

Step 3: Assess and Adjust Difficulty

- The therapist completes the Deliberate Practice Reaction Form (see Appendix A) and decides whether to make the exercise easier or harder or to repeat the same difficulty level.

Step 4: Repeat for Approximately 15 Minutes

- Repeat Steps 1 to 3 for at least 15 minutes.
- The trainees then switch therapist and client roles and start over.

Now it's your turn! Follow Steps 1 and 2 from the instructions.

Remember: The goal of the role play is for trainees to practice improvising responses to the client statements in a manner that (a) uses the skill criteria and (b) feels authentic for the trainee. **Example therapist responses for each client statement are provided at the end of this exercise. Trainees should attempt to improvise their own responses before reading the examples.**

BEGINNER CLIENT STATEMENTS FOR EXERCISE 10
Beginner Client Statement 1
[Upset] My roommate never washes up her dishes. She just leaves them in the sink or on the counter with such a look of innocence on her face like she doesn't know exactly what she's doing. I hate this; I have to do everything.
Beginner Client Statement 2
[Sad] I remember when my grandmother died. We were so close, and I was so lonely after that. I think my life really changed then. I was about 6 or 7.
Beginner Client Statement 3
[Tearfully] I can't believe my best friend is moving to Seattle. I am going to miss them so much.
Beginner Client Statement 4
[Scared, eyes wide open] I was so scared as a little boy. My father would fly into rages, and I would have to make sure my sisters and brothers were out of his way. It was awful.
Beginner Client Statement 5
[Happily smiling] My partner and I work so well together. It feels like we are a perfect team. They are amazing. I love them.

 Assess and adjust the difficulty before moving to the next difficulty level (see Step 3 in the exercise instructions).

INTERMEDIATE CLIENT STATEMENTS FOR EXERCISE 10
Intermediate Client Statement 1
[Regretfully] I wasn't the same after he assaulted me. Whenever he saw me, he always had this smirk on his face, and his life just went on as if nothing happened at all.
Intermediate Client Statement 2
[Tenderly] I can imagine my father as a little boy. His father was an alcoholic and abusive. I understand why he was so volatile toward me growing up.
Intermediate Client Statement 3
[Sadly] I really miss my friends from my hometown. I've been a bit weepy.
Intermediate Client Statement 4
[Wrinkling face with disgust] I feel nauseous even thinking about her. There is something about the way she never wears shoes. Her feet make me feel disgusted.
Intermediate Client Statement 5
[Thoughtful] My father never apologized to me. I think if he had, I would be able to get on with my life.

 Assess and adjust the difficulty before moving to the next difficulty level (see Step 3 in the exercise instructions).

ADVANCED CLIENT STATEMENTS FOR EXERCISE 10
Advanced Client Statement 1
[Fearful] My parents would fight all the time. My sister and I were always scared. I remember my sister's big eyes wide with fear when they'd be screaming at each other.
Advanced Client Statement 2
[Hopelessly, shoulders rounded, eyes downcast] My stepmother really hates me. She is turning my father against me. There is nothing I can do about it.
Advanced Client Statement 3
[Angrily] My partner shops all the time and treats himself to posh clothes. I don't know who he thinks he is. I would never spend money or wear fancy clothes like that.
Advanced Client Statement 4
[Shaking head in disbelief] When my partner talks to me like that, I feel disgusted. She has contempt for me. I don't even think she likes me.
Advanced Client Statement 5
[Tearfully] I feel so sad for myself when I think about how much I was alone, and yet I also feel really angry at my parents. They were a team, and I was always home with a sitter.

> **Assess and adjust the difficulty here (see Step 3 in the exercise instructions). If appropriate, follow the instructions to make the exercise even more challenging (see Appendix A).**

Example Therapist Responses: Initiating Portrayals

Remember: Trainees should attempt to improvise their own responses before reading the examples. **Do not read the following responses verbatim unless you are having trouble coming up with your own!**

EXAMPLE RESPONSES TO BEGINNER CLIENT STATEMENTS FOR EXERCISE 10
Example Response to Beginner Client Statement 1
So right here right now with me, if you imagined your roommate just leaving dishes on the counter or in the sink with that innocent look on her face, (Criterion 1) what would you want to say or do to her? (Criterion 2)
Example Response to Beginner Client Statement 2
So right here right now with me, if you imagine yourself at 6 or 7, (Criterion 1) what would you say or how would you be with that little child to let them know you get how lonely they were? (Criterion 2)
Example Response to Beginner Client Statement 3
So right here right now with me, if you imagine your best friend, (Criterion 1) and how you feel when you're with them, what would you want to say or do to let them know how much you are going to miss them? (Criterion 2)
Example Response to Beginner Client Statement 4
So right here right now with me, if you imagine yourself as a little boy protecting your brothers and sisters, (Criterion 1) what would you say or how would you be with him to comfort him and help him with his fear? (Criterion 2)
Example Response to Beginner Client Statement 5
So right here right now with me, if you imagine your partner (Criterion 1) and how you love them, (Criterion 1) what would you say to them to let them know? (Criterion 2)

EXAMPLE RESPONSES TO INTERMEDIATE CLIENT STATEMENTS FOR EXERCISE 10

Example Response to Intermediate Client Statement 1

So right here right now with me, if you imagine the man who assaulted you with that smirk on his face, (Criterion 1) what would you want to say or do to him to wipe that smirk off his face? (Criterion 2)

Example Response to Intermediate Client Statement 2

So right here, right now with me, if you imagine your father as a little boy, (Criterion 1) how would you be with him, and what would you say to him? (Criterion 2)

Example Response to Intermediate Client Statement 3

If you imagined your circle of friends with sad faces as you say good-bye, (Criterion 1) what would you say to let them know how much you miss them? (Criterion 2)

Example Response to Intermediate Client Statement 4

So right here right now with me, if you imagine her—and specifically her naked feet—(Criterion 1) what would happen if you really let this disgust out? (Criterion 2)

Example Response to Intermediate Client Statement 5

So right here right now with me, if you imagine your father, (Criterion 1) what would it feel like to let him know that you really needed an apology from him? (Criterion 2)

EXAMPLE RESPONSES TO ADVANCED CLIENT STATEMENTS FOR EXERCISE 10

Example Response to Advanced Client Statement 1

So right here right now with me, if you imagined your parents, (Criterion 1) what would you want to say or do to them to get them to stop? (Criterion 2)

or

If you conjured up your sister with her big wide eyes, (Criterion 1) how would you be with her and what would you say to her? (Criterion 2)

Example Response to Advanced Client Statement 2

So imagine your stepmother is right here with us, right now. (Criterion 1) What would you want to say or do to her about how she is turning your father against you? (Criterion 2)

Example Response to Advanced Client Statement 3

So right here with me, if you imagine your partner right now, (Criterion 1) what would you do or say to him directly? (Criterion 2)

Example Response to Advanced Client Statement 4

So right here with me, if you imagine your partner, (Criterion 1) what would you say to her? (Criterion 2)

Example Response to Advanced Client Statement 5

So right here right now with me, if you imagine your younger self, (Criterion 1) what would you want to say or do to let him know you get how lonely he felt? (Criterion 2)

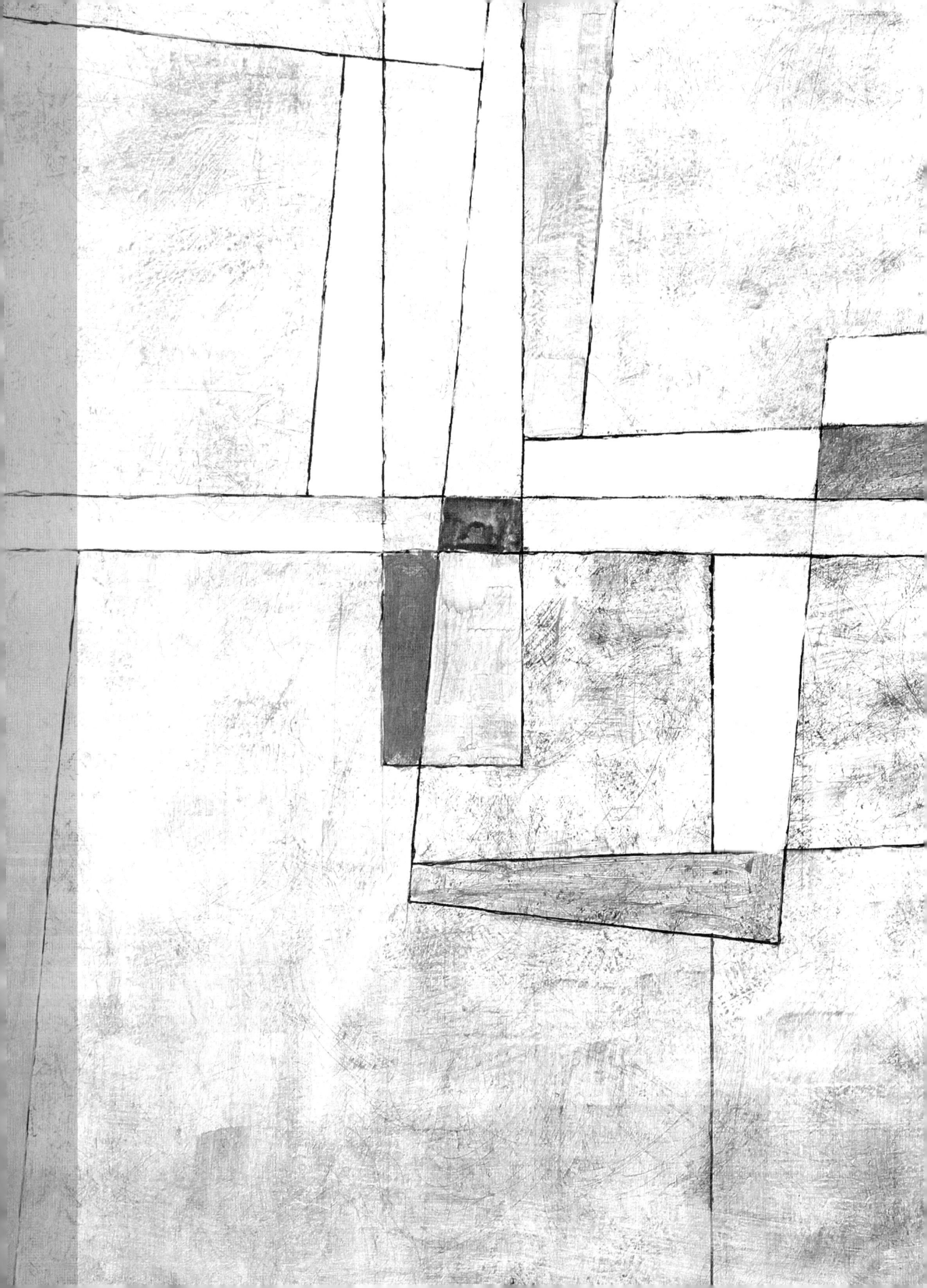

Privileging Transformance Strivings

Preparations for Exercise 11

1. Read the instructions in Chapter 2.

2. Download the Deliberate Practice Reaction Form and the Deliberate Practice Diary Form at https://www.apa.org/pubs/books/deliberate-practice-accelerated-experiential-dynamic-psychotherapy (see the "Resources" tab; also available in Appendixes A and B, respectively).

Skill Description

Skill Difficulty Level: Advanced

In accelerated experiential dynamic psychotherapy (AEDP), we use a particular way of attending to clients: We are "transformance detectives" which means that we are looking, feeling, tracking, and listening for glimmers of health, resilience, and strengths; exceptions to the established narrative of suffering or limitation; or a glimmer of being surprised by joy or possibility (K. Halliday, personal communication, 2023).

"Transformance" is an individual's innate drive to be transformed, to right oneself, to grow—to be authentic and be known, connected, and recognized by another. In AEDP, we try to set up conditions for transformance to come to the fore. From the very outset of therapy, we highlight the health the client already exhibits; this exercise takes that stance one step further as it focuses on the client's changing for the better—perhaps because of our efforts together.

Transformance is the opposite of resistance. It is the driving force inside all of us to self-right and lean toward health and healing. By highlighting strengths, we work to activate healing tendencies consistent with the broaden-and-build theory of positive

https://doi.org/10.1037/0000439-013

Deliberate Practice in Accelerated Experiential Dynamic Psychotherapy, by N. C. N. Prenn, H. Levenson, A. Vaz, and T. Rousmaniere

emotions (Fredrickson, 2001). In this skill, privileging transformance strivings, clinicians look for strengths that the client already has as well as glimmers of the client's moving in healthier directions.

The therapist's task is to improvise a response to each client statement following these skill criteria:

1. **Look and listen for opportunities to highlight where the client is saying or doing something healthier.** This first criterion falls under the rubric of the therapist's stance or attitude; it is an "internal" therapist skill (i.e., not an observable/verbal therapist behavior). We are on the lookout for shifts, change, an opening, or a glimmer of something new, different, and better.

2. **Use an AEDP skill from this book to celebrate, promote, or strengthen that healthier behavior.** You will be using skills you have already practiced in this book for various purposes, but this time you will use those skills to create an upward spiral of growth. You will find there are a number of AEDP skills that you can use to promote such positive change.

SKILL CRITERIA FOR EXERCISE 11

1. Look and listen for opportunities to highlight where the client is saying or doing something healthier.
2. Use an AEDP skill from this book to celebrate, promote, or strengthen that healthier behavior.

HELPFUL HINT

If for Criterion 2 you see yourself (or if your role-play partner sees you) favoring one skill over another, you might challenge yourself by trying less used skills, particularly as you progress to the advanced statements.

Examples of Therapists Privileging Transformance Strivings

Example 1

CLIENT: [*Soft*] As you know, I'm not usually this direct, but [voice trails off] . . . [stronger voice] well, if I'm really honest, [deep breath] when you asked me how I felt, the answer is, I really don't know.

THERAPIST: I am so glad you are being direct. I know it's hard for you. You are changing. That is great! (Criterion 2, Skill 4: Affirming)

or

I feel so much closer to you when you are so honest with me. (Criterion 2, Skill 5: Self-Involving Self-Disclosure)

or

I know from my own experience that it is not easy being direct. (Criterion 2, Skill 6: Self-Revealing Self-Disclosure)

Example 2

CLIENT: [*Nodding and smiling*] For the first time since before the promotion, I was able to give myself a break, take a nap, and delegate some of my work.

THERAPIST: That's so great that you delegated some of your work and took a nap. (Criterion 2, Skill 4: Affirming)

or

Good for you. I know how hard that can be personally to allow myself to take a nap. (Criterion 2, Skill 6: Self-Revealing Self-Disclosure)

Example 3

CLIENT: [*Angry*] I'm fed up with how my boss is treating me. I really need to address this with her at my next meeting.

THERAPIST: It's wonderful to hear you feeling assertive and wanting to speak up and address this. (Criterion 2, Skill 4: Affirming)

or

What does your body feel like as you say this? (Criterion 1, Skill 2: Exploring and Staying With Physical Experience)

or

I am so glad to hear this: I remember one of the first times I spoke up to my boss instead of just accepting not being treated well. (Criterion 2, Skill 5: Self-Involving Self-Disclosure)

INSTRUCTIONS FOR EXERCISE 11

Step 1: Role-Play and Feedback

- The client says the first beginner client statement. The therapist **improvises** a response based on the skill criteria.
- The trainer (or, if not available, the client) provides **brief** feedback based on the skill criteria.
- The client then repeats the same statement, and the therapist again improvises a response. The trainer (or client) again provides brief feedback.

Step 2: Repeat

- Repeat Step 1 for all the example statements **in the current difficulty level** (beginner, intermediate, or advanced).

Step 3: Assess and Adjust Difficulty

- The therapist completes the Deliberate Practice Reaction Form (see Appendix A) and decides whether to make the exercise easier or harder or to repeat the same difficulty level.

Step 4: Repeat for Approximately 15 Minutes

- Repeat Steps 1 to 3 for at least 15 minutes.
- The trainees then switch therapist and client roles and start over.

Now it's your turn! Follow Steps 1 and 2 from the instructions.

Remember: The goal of the role play is for trainees to practice improvising responses to the client statements in a manner that (a) uses the skill criteria and (b) feels authentic for the trainee. **Example therapist responses for each client statement are provided at the end of this exercise. Trainees should attempt to improvise their own responses before reading the examples.**

BEGINNER CLIENT STATEMENTS FOR EXERCISE 11
Beginner Client Statement 1
[Proud] As we talked about last week, I spoke up to my partner about one of those things that has been bothering me. It went really well. Much better than I expected.
Beginner Client Statement 2
[Happy] I feel good about being in therapy with you. [Shaking head in disbelief] Things are really changing, and I can't believe I look forward to coming to the sessions.
Beginner Client Statement 3
[Amazed] I noticed the old self-blaming voice coming up but I could also feel my anger. It's the first time I realized I'm angry and didn't blame myself.
Beginner Client Statement 4
[Proud] I felt so proud of myself when she said I had passed. I've wanted to get my driver's license for so long.
Beginner Client Statement 5
[With a big smile] As soon as I found out about the conference, I told my partner that I would be away. They appreciated that I looped them in immediately and didn't avoid telling them.

 Assess and adjust the difficulty before moving to the next difficulty level (see Step 3 in the exercise instructions).

INTERMEDIATE CLIENT STATEMENTS FOR EXERCISE 11

Intermediate Client Statement 1

[**Pleased with a big smile**] I was having a terrible day. The weather was so bad, and I was just feeling miserable. In the end, instead of my usual isolating, I called a friend, and we went to the gym together. I felt much better after that.

Intermediate Client Statement 2

[**Thoughtful**] I'm having a new experience right now. I can feel the sleepy defense coming over me, but I am aware of it and can feel myself choosing to stay with the anger toward my boss instead.

Intermediate Client Statement 3

[**Proud**] I spoke up to my partner over the weekend: We haven't been having sex, and I told them that it's important to me and we need to make it happen!

Intermediate Client Statement 4

[**Amazed**] Wow, I always feel anxious, and right now I don't feel any anxiety at all. This is weird!

Intermediate Client Statement 5

[**Happy**] I feel so pleased with myself: I felt that old negative voice come in after the interview went so well, but for the first time, I heard it distinctly and knew what it was: just a negative voice. I didn't let it ramp up, but just let myself feel proud that I had prepped thoroughly and it went super well.

 Assess and adjust the difficulty before moving to the next difficulty level (see Step 3 in the exercise instructions).

ADVANCED CLIENT STATEMENTS FOR EXERCISE 11
Advanced Client Statement 1
[Angry, make fists with hands] I felt angry with you last week: I felt like you were totally off with almost everything you said. I can feel I am still angry: I'm making fists with my hands as I'm sure you're noticing!
Advanced Client Statement 2
[Calm] I really felt good after last week's session. I felt so supported and close to you. [Make eye contact and then quickly look away] I feel embarrassed saying that.
Advanced Client Statement 3
[Serious] I nearly didn't come to the session today. I know I have missed coming in so many times before because I just don't feel up for anything, but today I forced myself to come.
Advanced Client Statement 4
[Surprised] I had such a good time with my friend. I can't believe it's possible to feel so close after the big fight we had.
Advanced Client Statement 5
[Big shy smile] I like seeing you every week. I'm really going to miss you while you're on vacation. Is that weird?

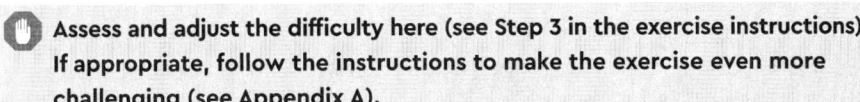 **Assess and adjust the difficulty here (see Step 3 in the exercise instructions). If appropriate, follow the instructions to make the exercise even more challenging (see Appendix A).**

Example Therapist Responses: Privileging Transformance Strivings

Remember: Trainees should attempt to improvise their own responses before reading the examples. **Do not read the following responses verbatim unless you are having trouble coming up with your own!**

EXAMPLE RESPONSES TO BEGINNER CLIENT STATEMENTS FOR EXERCISE 11
Example Response to Beginner Client Statement 1
It's wonderful to hear you speaking up and addressing things. (Criterion 2, Skill 4: Affirming)   or   I am so glad to hear this. I know how it can feel to speak up and not let things fester when something's bothering me. (Criterion 2, Skill 6: Self-Revealing Self-Disclosure)   or   When you spoke up, what was it like physically? (Criterion 1, Skill 2: Exploring and Staying With Physical Experience)
Example Response to Beginner Client Statement 2
I am delighted too. I look forward to our sessions too! (Criterion 2, Skill 5: Self-Involving Self-Disclosure)   or   Feel my delight with you as you say this. (Criterion 2, Skill 3: Undoing Aloneness)   or   When you are surprised that you look forward to therapy, what physical information does your body send you? (Criterion 1, Skill 2: Exploring and Staying With Physical Experience)
Example Response to Beginner Client Statement 3
It's wonderful to hear this change—you noticed your old way of being, and the new. This is a big deal. (Criterion 2, Skill 4: Affirming)   or   I am so glad to hear this; I know that personally too—the shift to "oh, wait, I'm angry and not blaming myself." (Criterion 2, Skill 6: Self-Revealing Self-Disclosure)   or   I'm so excited you were able to do that. (Criterion 2, Skill 5: Self-Involving Self-Disclosure)
Example Response to Beginner Client Statement 4
It's wonderful to hear that not only did you achieve this goal, but you also let yourself feel so proud. (Criterion 2, Skill 4: Affirming)   or   I am so glad to hear you felt so proud. I know how good letting myself feel proud can feel. (Criterion 2, Skill 6: Self-Revealing Self-Disclosure)   or   Feel me right alongside you as you say this. (Criterion 2, Skill 3: Undoing Aloneness)

EXAMPLE RESPONSES TO BEGINNER CLIENT STATEMENTS FOR EXERCISE 11
Example Response to Beginner Client Statement 5
It's wonderful to hear you being proactive. (Criterion 2, Skill 4: Affirming) or I am so glad to hear this. I know how it can feel to speak up and not put off telling somebody something they won't be pleased to hear (Criterion 2, Skill 6: Self-Revealing Self-Disclosure) or I had a sense you'd be able to speak up; what did that feel like inside physically? (Criterion 1, Skill 2: Exploring and Staying With Physical Experience)

EXAMPLE RESPONSES TO INTERMEDIATE CLIENT STATEMENTS FOR EXERCISE 11

Example Response to Intermediate Client Statement 1

Good for you for figuring out what you needed on a rainy day and doing something different. (Criterion 2, Skill 4: Affirming)

or

What does it feel like inside your body sharing with me that you did something different? (Criterion 1, Skill 2: Exploring and Staying With Physical Experience)

or

That is such a big smile as you tell me this. (Criterion 2, Skill 1: Moment-to-Moment Tracking)

Example Response to Intermediate Client Statement 2

It is so growthful that you can feel that choice. (Criterion 2, Skill 4: Affirming)

or

What is it like physically in your body to make that choice? (Criterion 1, Skill 2: Exploring and Staying With Physical Experience)

or

Feel me with you as you feel that. (Criterion 2, Skill 3: Undoing Aloneness)

Example Response to Intermediate Client Statement 3

I feel proud of you hearing you being assertive and stating your needs. (Criterion 2, Skill 5: Self-Involving Self-Disclosure)

or

What is it like physically to be so direct like that? (Criterion 1, Skill 2: Exploring and Staying With Physical Experience)

or

Feel me with you as you feel that. (Criterion 2, Skill 3: Undoing Aloneness)

Example Response to Intermediate Client Statement 4

It is so great that you notice that. (Criterion 2, Skill 4: Affirming)

or

Wow! What's your body feel like when it is not anxious? (Criterion 1, Skill 2: Exploring and Staying With Physical Experience)

or

Feel me with you as you feel this new experience of no anxiety. (Criterion 2, Skill 3: Undoing Aloneness)

Example Response to Intermediate Client Statement 5

I feel so happy with you—that you could let yourself feel pleased and not go that old negative voice. (Criterion 2, Skill 5: Self-Involving Self-Disclosure)

or

What is it like sharing with me right now that you had such a different experience? (Criterion 2, Skill 7: Metaprocessing)

or

Stay with the physical feeling of being pleased with yourself. (Criterion 2, Skill 2: Exploring and Staying With Physical Experience)

EXAMPLE RESPONSES TO ADVANCED CLIENT STATEMENTS FOR EXERCISE 11

Example Response to Advanced Client Statement 1

What do your fists want to say, if you let them speak? (Criterion 2, Skill 10: Initiating Portrayals)

or

Can you stay with the physical energy of the anger? This is important. (Criterion 2, Skill 2: Exploring and Staying With Physical Experience)

or

It may sound like a funny thing to say, but I feel connected to you right now because your anger feels authentic and right on. (Criterion 2, Skill 5: Self-Involving Self-Disclosure)

Example Response to Advanced Client Statement 2

I am so glad you felt supported and close to me. And what would happen if you didn't look away, which probably helped your nervous system growing up, but instead right now looked my way again? (Criterion 2, Skill 9: Affirmative Work With Defenses)

or

Feel me with you as you feel that embarrassment. I am so glad you feel close and supported by me. (Criterion 2, Skill 3: Undoing Aloneness)

or

From this place of closeness and support, what would you want to say to me? (Criterion 2, Skill 10: Initiating Portrayals)

Example Response to Advanced Client Statement 3

I'm so glad you came into session and that you are letting me know how you don't feel up for anything right now. (Criterion 2, Skill 4: Affirming)

or

It is so important that you feel me with you as you say this and that you're not alone with this. (Criterion 2, Skill 3: Undoing Aloneness)

or

It speaks to your determination to get better. It makes me hopeful about our work together. (Criterion 2, Skill 6: Self-Revealing Self-Disclosure)

Example Response to Advanced Client Statement 4

I've had that realization too—learning that speaking up and having a fight can ultimately make people closer. (Criterion 2, Skill 6: Self-Revealing Self-Disclosure)

or

Can we just stay with the physical experience of surprise at something new? (Criterion 2, Skill 2: Exploring and Staying With Physical Experience)

or

This is a big change! You have worked hard to try new things, and it is growing your capacity. (Criterion 2, Skill 4: Affirming)

EXAMPLE RESPONSES TO ADVANCED CLIENT STATEMENTS FOR EXERCISE 11

Example Response to Advanced Client Statement 5

It isn't weird that you'll miss me. We're deeply connected, you and I. I'm so glad you like seeing me every week. I look forward to our sessions too. (Criterion 2, Skill 5: Self-Involving Self-Disclosure)

or

No, it's healthy! And would it be okay with you if we stayed with this big shy smile and just notice what that's like inside, physically. (Criterion 2, Skill 2: Exploring and Staying With Physical Experience)

or

No, it is a good thing. Feel me with you as you feel that. (Criterion 2, Skill 3: Undoing Aloneness)

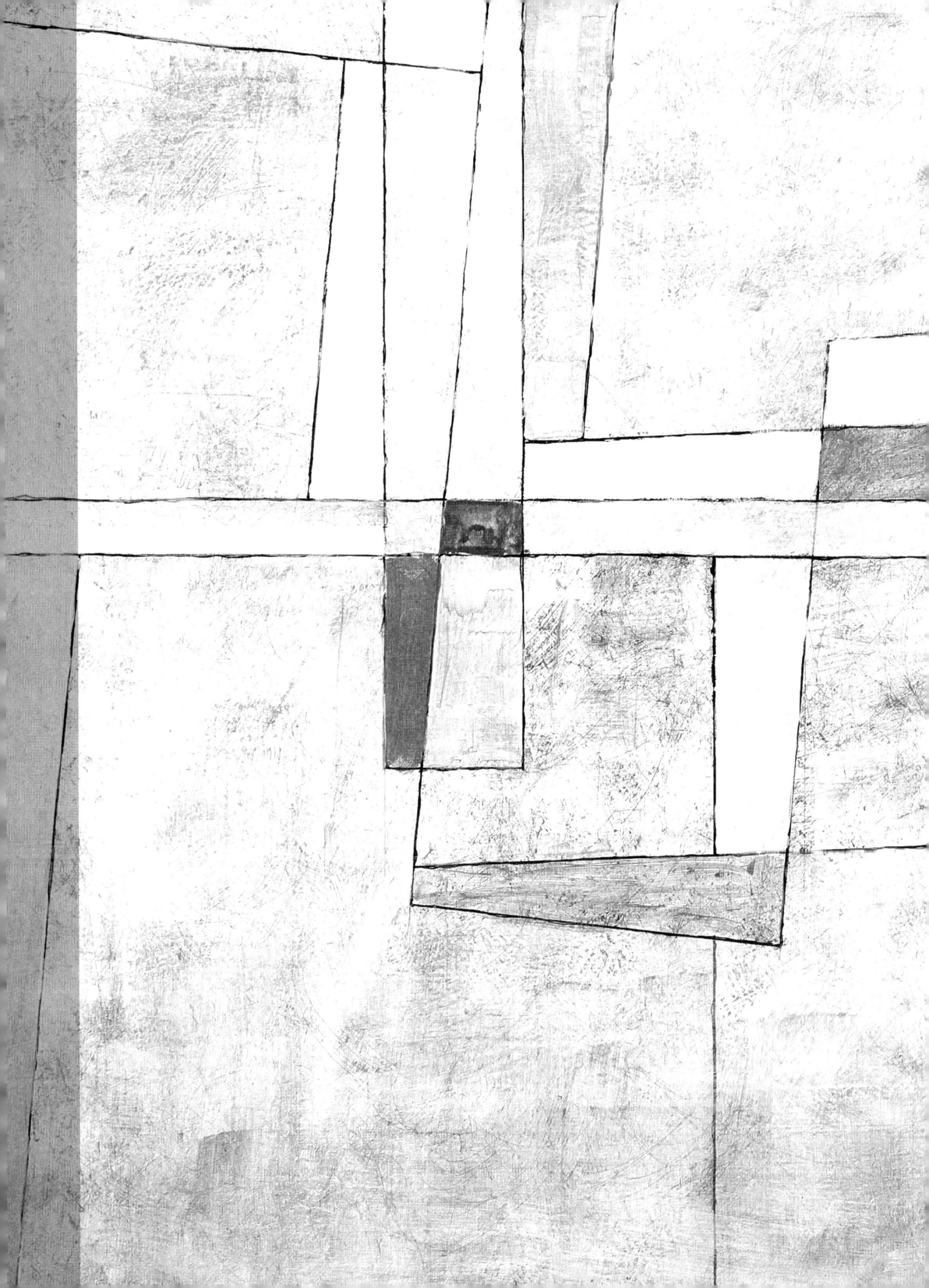

Metatherapeutic Processing

Preparations for Exercise 12

1. Read the instructions in Chapter 2.

2. Download the Deliberate Practice Reaction Form and the Deliberate Practice Diary Form at https://www.apa.org/pubs/books/deliberate-practice-accelerated-experiential-dynamic-psychotherapy (see the "Resources" tab; also available in Appendixes A and B, respectively).

Skill Description

Skill Difficulty Level: Advanced

In accelerated experiential dynamic psychotherapy (AEDP), metatherapeutic processing is an emotional (within) and relational (between) exploratory process focusing on the client's *experience of change for the better* (Fosha, 2009, 2021; Fosha & Thoma, 2020). It is a skill that focuses on processing the experience of what is therapeutic about therapy. In this way, metatherapeutic processing is a reflecting skill that harnesses and anchors growth and change for the better. The rationale behind metatherapeutic processing is that we not only learn from experience; we learn from reflecting on that experience. What is often an endpoint in other therapies is a starting point in AEDP. We process and explore growth and positive change as thoroughly as psychotherapy has traditionally explored pathology.

Metatherapeutic processing can be an *exploration of an internal, somatic experience* of change for the better such as, "So you're saying that you're feeling better. And you have a sense that maybe you can be more effective. What does it feel like inside to have that sense of being more effective?" Or metatherapeutic processing can be the *processing of a growthful, relational experience* such as, "What's it like that you and I, through talking together and doing this piece of work together, are now having

https://doi.org/10.1037/0000439-014

Deliberate Practice in Accelerated Experiential Dynamic Psychotherapy, by N. C. N. Prenn, H. Levenson, A. Vaz, and T. Rousmaniere

this experience of mastery [or mourning or feeling better]?" (D. Fosha, 2016, personal communication). The goal for both the internal and relational approaches is to help clients reflect on and take in the positive experience.

Metatherapeutic processing is a type of reflection, but we keep it experiential by focusing on the exploration of the new experience both somatically and interpersonally. This bottom-up approach allows new realizations as beliefs or cognitions to come to the fore. It also deepens the client's emotional experience of the change for the better, as the exploration promotes further access to and expanding of the client's feelings, triggering a self-perpetuating upward spiral. In addition, research indicates that focusing on such positive emotions appears to have an overall beneficial effect on the working alliance (Notsu et al., 2023).

The therapist's task is to improvise a response to each client statement following these skill criteria:

1. **Ask the client an open-ended question about a positive shift or change for the better that they have mentioned.** The shift or change can be internal or interpersonal. It can be a brief piece of work within a session or reflecting on the whole session or series of sessions. The most important thing is to notice and seize markers and expressions of transformation. After doing this, wait for the person playing the client to reply with their scripted statement. Then proceed to the next skill criterion.

2. **Continue to ask open-ended questions focusing on deepening the client's experience of change for the better.** Metatherapeutic processing is a process. Think of it as a positive spiral that builds on itself using the standard question, "What is *that* like?" followed by "And what is *that* like?" The therapist focuses on whatever emerges in the just completed round of exploration and deepening. In the clinical setting, this process would continue for as long as new experiences of therapeutic change continue to unfold. For this exercise, we will only do two cycles. Because we are engaging in an ongoing back and forth with clients in this exercise, the exercise takes a dialogue format.

<table>
<tr><td colspan="2">SKILL CRITERIA FOR EXERCISE 12</td></tr>
<tr><td>1.</td><td>Ask the client an open-ended question about a positive shift or change for the better that they have mentioned.</td></tr>
<tr><td>2.</td><td>Continue to ask open-ended questions focusing on exploring and deepening the client's experience of change for the better.</td></tr>
</table>

<table>
<tr><td colspan="2">HELPFUL HINTS</td></tr>
<tr><td>1.</td><td>When you ask open-ended questions following up on the client's experience, try not to say something vague such as, "And what's that like?" Rather ground the question in the specifics of what the client has just said whenever possible: "And what does that warmth feel like?"</td></tr>
<tr><td>2.</td><td>After successful completion of the first two beginner dialogues, the therapist can try doing the exercise without the therapist prompts being read.</td></tr>
</table>

Example of a Therapist Using Metatherapeutic Processing

Example

CLIENT: [*Proud*] That was an amazing session! I can't believe how relieved I'm feeling!

THERAPIST: What's it like that we had this amazing session today? (Criterion 1)

CLIENT: [*Puzzled*] I'm kind of surprised that it actually feels great! [*Smiling*] I feel a kind of internal warmth.

THERAPIST: And what does that warmth feel like? (Criterion 2)

CLIENT: [*Smiling broadly*] I guess . . . it's like there's this beam of light shining from my body.

THERAPIST: And what's that light shining from your body feel like? (Criterion 2)

CLIENT: [*Excited*] It's like I'm alive for the first time in my life!

INSTRUCTIONS FOR EXERCISE 12

Step 1: Role-Play and Feedback

- The client initiates the dialogue by reading the first statement in the beginner dialogue and reads the therapist prompt. Then the therapist **improvises** a response following the first skill criterion.
- The client reads the next statement in the same dialogue followed by the therapist prompt for Criterion 2, and the therapist improvises a response. This continues until the dialogue has been completed.
- The trainer (or, if not available, the client) provides **brief** feedback based on the skill criteria.
- The client and the therapist then repeat the same dialogue with the therapist again improvising responses. The trainer (or client) again provides brief feedback.

Step 2: Repeat

- Repeat Step 1 for all the dialogues **in the current difficulty level** (beginner, intermediate, or advanced).

Step 3: Assess and Adjust Difficulty

- The therapist completes the Deliberate Practice Reaction Form (see Appendix A) and decides whether to make the exercise easier or harder or to repeat the same difficulty level.

Step 4: Repeat for Approximately 15 Minutes

- Repeat Steps 1 to 3 for at least 15 minutes.
- The trainees then switch therapist and client roles and start over.

> **Now it's your turn! Follow Steps 1 and 2 from the instructions.**

Remember: The goal of the role play is for trainees to practice improvising responses to the client statements in a manner that (a) uses the skill criteria and (b) feels authentic for the trainee. **Example therapist responses for each client statement are provided at the end of this exercise. Trainees should attempt to improvise their own responses before reading the examples.**

BEGINNER DIALOGUE 1
CLIENT: [Excited] Huh. Wow! Right now, I'm suddenly aware of how I feel much better. Wow! [Grins]
THERAPIST PROMPT (CRITERION 1): Ask the client an open-ended question about a positive shift or change for the better that they have mentioned.
CLIENT: [Smiling broadly] I'm kind of surprised that it actually feels great! I feel a kind of warmth inside.
THERAPIST PROMPT (CRITERION 2): Continue to ask open-ended questions focusing on exploring and deepening the client's experience of change for the better.
CLIENT: [Curious] It's really expansive—like I can breathe more easily.
THERAPIST PROMPT (CRITERION 2): Continue to ask open-ended questions focusing on exploring and deepening the client's experience of change for the better.
CLIENT: [Delighted] It's like I've got a new lease on life.

BEGINNER DIALOGUE 2
CLIENT: **[Proud]** I think last week's session shifted something in me. I had such a good week. I felt more confident and was able to speak up. It felt really different.
THERAPIST PROMPT (CRITERION 1): Ask the client an open-ended question about a positive shift or change for the better that they have mentioned.
CLIENT: **[Surprised]** I'm kind of surprised that therapy works. I didn't expect that.
THERAPIST PROMPT (CRITERION 2): Continue to ask open-ended questions focusing on exploring and deepening the client's experience of change for the better.
CLIENT: **[Beaming]** It's great. It feels good.
THERAPIST PROMPT (CRITERION 2): Continue to ask open-ended questions focusing on exploring and deepening the client's experience of change for the better.
CLIENT: **[Sitting upright]** Kind of amazing. Warm and like I have a straighter spine.

BEGINNER DIALOGUE 3
CLIENT: [Surprised] Huh. Wow! I'm so glad I finally told you about that. I feel like it took a weight off!
THERAPIST PROMPT (CRITERION 1): Ask the client an open-ended question about a positive shift or change for the better that they have mentioned.
CLIENT: [Smiling] So much lighter. . . . Wow! Thank you.
THERAPIST PROMPT (CRITERION 2): Continue to ask open-ended questions focusing on exploring and deepening the client's experience of change for the better.
CLIENT: [Taking a deep breath] I feel like I can breathe again . . . like my chest can fill with air again.
THERAPIST PROMPT (CRITERION 2): Continue to ask open-ended questions focusing on exploring and deepening the client's experience of change for the better.
CLIENT: [Puzzled] It feels weird, new, different actually. Like I can actually breathe the right way!

BEGINNER DIALOGUE 4
CLIENT: **[Surprised]** Wow, I always feel anxious, and right now, after going through all this painful stuff with you, I don't feel any anxiety at all.
THERAPIST PROMPT (CRITERION 1): Ask the client an open-ended question about a positive shift or change for the better that they have mentioned.
CLIENT: **[Calm]** It's weird. I feel calm.
THERAPIST PROMPT (CRITERION 2): Continue to ask open-ended questions focusing on exploring and deepening the client's experience of change for the better.
CLIENT: **[Taking in and letting out a deep breath]** It's like my shoulders aren't up around my ears . . . like a big exhale.
THERAPIST PROMPT (CRITERION 2): Continue to ask open-ended questions focusing on exploring and deepening the client's experience of change for the better.
CLIENT: **[Peaceful]** It feels like hope like I can actually change.

🖐 **Assess and adjust the difficulty before moving to the next difficulty level (see Step 3 in the exercise instructions).**

INTERMEDIATE DIALOGUE 1
CLIENT: **[Thoughtful]** I kept hearing your voice encouraging me. And hearing your voice really helped me move forward.
THERAPIST PROMPT (CRITERION 1): Ask the client an open-ended question about a positive shift or change for the better that they have mentioned.
CLIENT: **[Smiling]** It was nice. A very different experience.
THERAPIST PROMPT (CRITERION 2): Continue to ask open-ended questions focusing on exploring and deepening the client's experience of change for the better.
CLIENT: **[Thoughtful and slow]** It's great. It feels good. I don't feel so alone.
THERAPIST PROMPT (CRITERION 2): Continue to ask open-ended questions focusing on exploring and deepening the client's experience of change for the better.
CLIENT: **[Delighted]** Inside . . . physically, it feels reassuring, like I can move forward in my life!

INTERMEDIATE DIALOGUE 2
CLIENT: **[Surprised]** Looking back to our first session and your saying you knew I would get through this made all the difference to me. You said I'd feel differently over time, and I do.
THERAPIST PROMPT (CRITERION 1): Ask the client an open-ended question about a positive shift or change for the better that they have mentioned.
CLIENT: **[Smiling]** It brings such an amazed smile to my insides.
THERAPIST PROMPT (CRITERION 2): Continue to ask open-ended questions focusing on exploring and deepening the client's experience of change for the better.
CLIENT: **[Surprised]** I feel like there is more space between my ribs and my hips, if that makes sense.
THERAPIST PROMPT (CRITERION 2): Continue to ask open-ended questions focusing on exploring and deepening the client's experience of change for the better.
CLIENT: **[Amazed]** It feels new and great and like I'm in touch with a superpower that I can be helped and that things do change. I didn't know that before. I thought I would feel upside down forever.

INTERMEDIATE DIALOGUE 3
CLIENT: [Proud] I used to just blame myself and feel guilty whenever my partner and I disagreed, but last week I had such a sense that she wasn't being fair; I was angry maybe for the first time in my life!
THERAPIST PROMPT (CRITERION 1): Ask the client an open-ended question about a positive shift or change for the better that they have mentioned.
CLIENT: [Straightforward] It was like I had a choice, and I could see it—blame myself or be angry. And I could see the choice right there!
THERAPIST PROMPT (CRITERION 2): Continue to ask open-ended questions focusing on exploring and deepening the client's experience of change for the better.
CLIENT: [Energetic] It was almost scary at first but then exciting, actually.
THERAPIST PROMPT (CRITERION 2): Continue to ask open-ended questions focusing on exploring and deepening the client's experience of change for the better.
CLIENT: [Knowing] It's powerful, like I can fight for myself instead of retreating and feeling bad.

 Assess and adjust the difficulty before moving to the next difficulty level (see Step 3 in the exercise instructions).

ADVANCED DIALOGUE 1
CLIENT: **[Excited]** I love all we are doing together. In other therapies I've been in, we talk about what we can do or might do in the future, but I feel that we are just doing it right now!
THERAPIST PROMPT (CRITERION 1): Ask the client an open-ended question about a positive shift or change for the better that they have mentioned.
CLIENT: **[Calm]** It is different. I now know that I can change and be on a team.
THERAPIST PROMPT (CRITERION 2): Continue to ask open-ended questions focusing on exploring and deepening the client's experience of change for the better.
CLIENT: **[Happy]** It's great. It feels good. I feel sort of clear-eyed, if that makes sense.
THERAPIST PROMPT (CRITERION 2): Continue to ask open-ended questions focusing on exploring and deepening the client's experience of change for the better.
CLIENT: **[Surprised]** It's bright and light and oddly sort of wise.

ADVANCED DIALOGUE 2
CLIENT: [Surprised] I feel that you really get me. I wonder if you have been through something similar.
THERAPIST PROMPT (CRITERION 1): Ask the client an open-ended question about a positive shift or change for the better that they have mentioned.
CLIENT: [Delighted] It feels warm and fuzzy in my heart.
THERAPIST PROMPT (CRITERION 2): Continue to ask open-ended questions focusing on exploring and deepening the client's experience of change for the better.
CLIENT: [Coherent] I feel like a powerful force is melting my ice barrier.
THERAPIST PROMPT (CRITERION 2): Continue to ask open-ended questions focusing on exploring and deepening the client's experience of change for the better.
CLIENT: [Ecstatic] Like freedom—like I can swim out into the ocean. Like I'm almost free!

ADVANCED DIALOGUE 3
CLIENT: [Straightforward] You know I have a hard time expressing anger. Well, I realize now I was angry with you last week. I didn't feel like you were getting me and you seemed to be just giving me advice. [Pause] And somehow I'm aware it's good that I felt angry.
THERAPIST PROMPT (CRITERION 1): Ask the client an open-ended question about a positive shift or change for the better that they have mentioned.
CLIENT: [Thoughtful] It was scary. It is scary—but it's a good-scary.
THERAPIST PROMPT (CRITERION 2): Continue to ask open-ended questions focusing on exploring and deepening the client's experience of change for the better.
CLIENT: [Puzzled] It's a new awareness. I don't think I have let myself be angry in that way before. I'm surprised it feels good.
THERAPIST PROMPT (CRITERION 2): Continue to ask open-ended questions focusing on exploring and deepening the client's experience of change for the better.
CLIENT: [Relaxed] It's good, new, different—like oh, this is what you meant about feelings. It isn't destroying our relationship. Weirdly, it's making me feel closer to you, if that makes sense.

 Assess and adjust the difficulty here (see Step 3 in the exercise instructions). If appropriate, follow the instructions to make the exercise even more challenging (see Appendix A).

Example Therapist Responses: Metatherapeutic Processing

Remember: Trainees should attempt to improvise their own responses before reading the examples. **Do not read the following responses verbatim unless you are having trouble coming up with your own!**

EXAMPLE THERAPIST RESPONSES FOR BEGINNER DIALOGUE 1
CLIENT: [Excited] Huh. Wow! Right now I'm suddenly aware of how I feel much better. Wow! [Grins]
THERAPIST: Wow . . . what's the "much better" like inside?
CLIENT: [Smiling broadly] I'm kind of surprised that it actually feels great! I feel a kind of warmth inside.
THERAPIST: Oh wow! And what's the warmth inside physically like?
CLIENT: [Curious] It's really expansive—like I can breathe more easily.
THERAPIST: And what's the expansive breathing like?
CLIENT: [Delighted] It's like I've got a new lease on life.

EXAMPLE THERAPIST RESPONSES FOR BEGINNER DIALOGUE 2
CLIENT: [Proud] I think last week's session shifted something in me. I had such a good week—I felt more confident and was able to speak up. It felt really different.
THERAPIST: What's it like that last week's session shifted something inside of you?
CLIENT: [Surprised] I'm kind of surprised. . . . Therapy works. I didn't expect that.
THERAPIST: Oh wow! And what's it like to say the therapy is working?
CLIENT: [Beaming] It's great. It feels good.
THERAPIST: And . . . inside, what's the good like?
CLIENT: [Sitting upright] Kind of amazing. Warm and like I have a straighter spine.

EXAMPLE THERAPIST RESPONSES FOR BEGINNER DIALOGUE 3
CLIENT: [Surprised] Huh. Wow. I'm so glad I finally told you about that. I feel like it took a weight off!
THERAPIST: What's it like having that weight off?
CLIENT: [Smiling] So much lighter . . . wow! Thank you.
THERAPIST: [Smiling and nodding back] You're welcome. What's it like, the "much lighter"?
CLIENT: [Taking a deep breath] I feel like I can breathe again . . . like my chest can fill with air again.
THERAPIST: And how does that feel inside when your chest fills with air!?
CLIENT: [Puzzled] It's feels weird, new, different, actually. Like I can actually breathe the right way!

EXAMPLE THERAPIST RESPONSES FOR BEGINNER DIALOGUE 4
CLIENT: [Surprised] Wow, I always feel anxious, and right now I don't feel any anxiety at all.
THERAPIST: How is that physically [pause] not feeling any anxiety?
CLIENT: [Calm] It's weird. I feel calm.
THERAPIST: What's the calm like?
CLIENT: [Taking in and letting out a deep breath] It's like my shoulders aren't up around my ears . . . like a big exhale.
THERAPIST: And how does that feel—the big exhale?
CLIENT: [Peaceful] It feels like hope—like I can actually change.

EXAMPLE THERAPIST RESPONSES FOR INTERMEDIATE DIALOGUE 1
CLIENT: **[Thoughtful]** I kept hearing your voice encouraging me. And hearing your voice really helped me move forward.
THERAPIST: What was that like for you to hear my voice with you?
CLIENT: **[Smiling]** It was nice. A very different experience.
THERAPIST: So what's it like that I am helping you?
CLIENT: **[Thoughtful and slow]** It's great. It feels good. I don't feel so alone.
THERAPIST: And . . . physically inside what's the "not so alone" like?
CLIENT: **[Delighted]** Inside . . . physically, it feels reassuring like I can move forward with my life!

EXAMPLE THERAPIST RESPONSES FOR INTERMEDIATE DIALOGUE 2
CLIENT: [Surprised] Looking back to our first session and your saying you knew I would get through this made all the difference to me. You said I'd feel differently over time, and I do.
THERAPIST: What's that like to remember my saying that to you?
CLIENT: [Smiling] It brings such an amazed smile to my insides.
THERAPIST: Oh, I love that! How does the amazed smile feel physically to your insides?
CLIENT: [Surprised] I feel like there is more space between my ribs and my hips, if that makes sense.
THERAPIST: It makes perfect sense! And what's that space like right now?
CLIENT: [Amazed] It feels new and great and like I'm in touch with a superpower that I can be helped and that things do change. I didn't know that before. I thought I would feel upside down forever.

EXAMPLE THERAPIST RESPONSES FOR INTERMEDIATE DIALOGUE 3
CLIENT: **[Proud]** I used to just blame myself and feel guilty whenever my partner and I disagreed, but last week I had such a sense that she wasn't being fair; I was angry maybe for the first time in my life!
THERAPIST: Wow! What was it like to feel that anger come up instead of self-blame?
CLIENT: **[Straightforward]** It was like I had a choice, and I could see it—blame myself or be angry. And I could see the choice right there!
THERAPIST: And what was that like to see the choice right there?
CLIENT: **[Energetic]** It was almost scary at first but then exciting, actually.
THERAPIST: And tell me what is that excitement like?
CLIENT: **[Knowing]** It's powerful, like I can fight for myself instead of retreating and feeling bad.

EXAMPLE THERAPIST RESPONSES FOR ADVANCED DIALOGUE 1
CLIENT: **[Excited]** I love all we are doing together. In other therapies I've been in, we talk about what we can do or might do in the future, but I feel that we are just doing it right now!
THERAPIST: What is it like to feel we are doing it and that you are loving it?
CLIENT: **[Calm]** It is different. I now know that I can change and be on a team.
THERAPIST: So what's it feel like inside of you that I am helping you and we're a team?
CLIENT: **[Happy]** It's great. It feels good. I feel sort of clear-eyed, if that makes sense.
THERAPIST: It makes perfect sense. And . . . physically, what's the clear-eyed like?
CLIENT: **[Surprised]** It's bright and light and oddly sort of grown up.

EXAMPLE THERAPIST RESPONSES FOR ADVANCED DIALOGUE 2
CLIENT: **[Surprised]** I feel that you really get me. I wonder if you have been through something similar.
THERAPIST: What's that like, to feel I really get you and that I may have gone through something similar?
CLIENT: **[Delighted]** It feels warm and fuzzy in my heart.
THERAPIST: Oh, I love that! What's the warm and fuzzy around your heart like sensation-wise?
CLIENT: **[Coherent]** I feel like a powerful force is melting my ice barrier.
THERAPIST: And what's that melting like right now?
CLIENT: **[Ecstatic]** Like freedom—like I can swim out into the ocean. Like I'm almost free!

EXAMPLE THERAPIST RESPONSES FOR ADVANCED DIALOGUE 3
CLIENT: [Straightforward] You know I have a hard time expressing anger. Well, I realize now I was angry with you last week. I didn't feel like you were getting me, and you seemed to be just giving me advice. [Pause] And somehow I'm aware it's good that I felt angry.
THERAPIST: I am so glad you are telling me. What is it like inside to realize that somehow it's good that you were angry?
CLIENT: [Thoughtful] It was scary. It is scary—but it's a good-scary.
THERAPIST: And what is that like to notice it's good-scary?
CLIENT: [Puzzled] It's a new awareness. I don't think I have let myself be angry in that way before. I'm surprised it feels good.
THERAPIST: And what's that surprise like?
CLIENT: [Relaxed] It's good, new, different—like oh, this is what you meant about feelings. It isn't destroying our relationship. Weirdly, it's making me feel closer to you, if that makes sense.

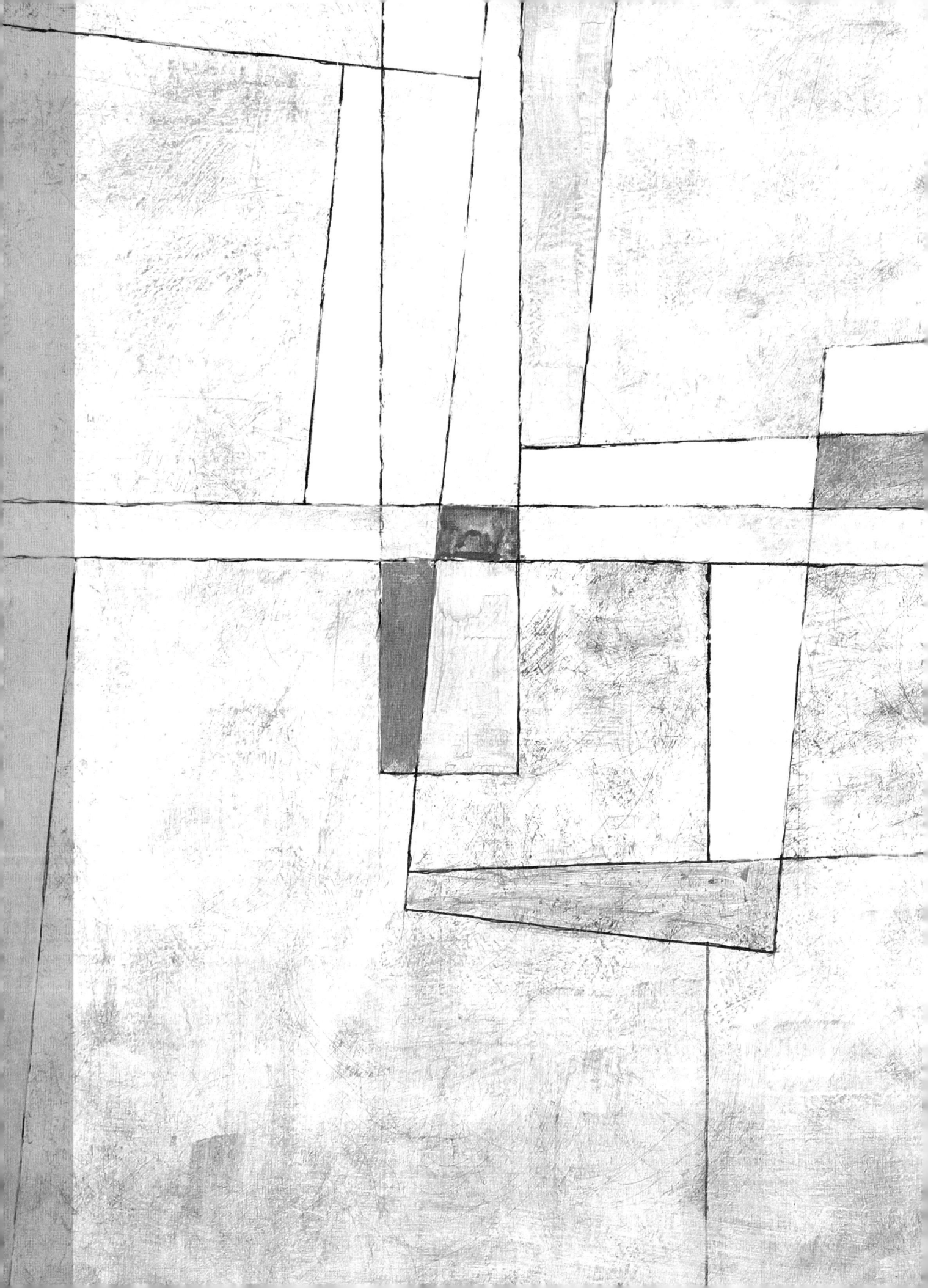

Annotated Accelerated Experiential Dynamic Psychotherapy Practice Session Transcript

It is now time to put all the skills you have learned together! Each therapist statement is annotated to indicate which accelerated experiential dynamic psychotherapy (AEDP) skill from Exercises 1 through 12 is used. This transcript provides an example of how therapists can interweave many AEDP skills in response to clients.

Instructions

As in the previous exercises, one trainee can play the client while the other plays the therapist. As much as possible, the trainee who plays the client should try to adopt an authentic emotional tone as if they are a real client. Both participants can read line-by-line from the transcript. As with all deliberate practice, try it once and then try it again! The purpose of this transcript is to provide you with an opportunity to experience how it feels to offer all the AEDP skills in the context of a session, albeit condensed, that mimics live therapy.

Note to Therapists

Remember to be aware of your vocal quality. Match your tone to the client's presentation. Thus, if the clients present vulnerable, soft emotions behind their words, soften your tone to be soothing and calm. If clients on the other hand, are aggressive and angry, match your tone to be firm and solid.

https://doi.org/10.1037/0000439-015

Deliberate Practice in Accelerated Experiential Dynamic Psychotherapy, by N. C. N. Prenn, H. Levenson, A. Vaz, and T. Rousmaniere

Annotated Accelerated Experiential Dynamic Psychotherapy Transcript

CLIENT 1: I was with my dad for dinner last night. We had a nice time, I guess. [Slaps thigh and laughs]

THERAPIST 1: A nice time with your dad, and you laugh and slap your thigh. (Skill 1: Moment-to Moment Tracking)

CLIENT 2: Yeah, it was a "nice" time although you know he always treats the wait staff so badly, and last night was no exception. He was rude. It was embarrassing. [Smiles and tucks hands under armpits]

THERAPIST 2: He was rude, and you smile and tuck your hands under your arms. (Skill 1: Moment-to-Moment Tracking) [Tucks hands under arms] Hard to have negative feelings toward him. (Skill 9: Affirmative Work With Defenses) What does it feel like physically to say he's rude? (Skill 2: Exploring and Staying With Physical Experience)

CLIENT 3: Ugh, he's such a bad person! He's a terrible person. [Rounds shoulders and slumps with hands still tucked under armpits]

THERAPIST 3: He is a terrible person. You have told me specifics. He can be really terrible. And he is rude, and you feel embarrassed. What's that feel like in your body? What do you notice? (Skill 2: Exploring and Staying With Physical Experience)

CLIENT 4: Ugh. I don't know. A weight on my shoulders. I find it difficult to get a full breath. I feel hopeless.

THERAPIST 4: I get that and I sense that. You round your shoulders and hunch over. (Skill 1: Moment-to-Moment Tracking) What would it be like to sit up straight and tell him directly how you feel? (Skill 10: Initiating Portrayals)

CLIENT 5: I'm sitting here and my life is such a mess. I can't do anything. I'm riddled with anxiety and immobility and it's his fault. He terrorized me, and I'm haunted by him.

THERAPIST 5: You feel it now that anxiety and immobility? (Skill 8: Working With Anxiety)

CLIENT 6: I do. I feel all sweaty and breathless and like my heart is jumping right through my ribs.

THERAPIST 6: Does it feel manageable, the anxiety? (Skill 8: Working With Anxiety)

CLIENT 7: It does. It does. But I'm really feeling it.

THERAPIST 7: That's great you notice it and feel it. (Skill 4: Affirming) And, as you know, anxiety lets us both know you're having big feelings. So, if you can let yourself notice it, what's coming up?

CLIENT 8: I don't know. I don't know. I just hate him. [Tucks hands tighter into armpits]

THERAPIST 8: Right. Right. I know. I know. And so right here with me, if you untucked your arms, sat up straight, and feel me with you here to help, (Skill 3: Undoing Aloneness) what would you want to say and do to him directly to let him know how you feel? And he's not here and will never know. This is just for us and for you to know how you feel. (Skill 10: Initiating Portrayals)

CLIENT 9: [He sits up straight] Ah, he just screwed me. All of this is his fault. It's his fucking fault.

THERAPIST 9: Yeah. So feel me with you, (Skill 3: Undoing Aloneness) and I feel mad at him too. (Skill 5: Self-Involving Self-Disclosure) See him here [pointing at nearby chair]. Tell him, "This is your fault." I'd like you to imagine him right here. What do you call him? Do you call him "Dad"? What do you call him? (Skill 10: Initiating Portrayals)

CLIENT 10: Ugh . . . Dad, I guess. Alright, I'll try. I hate doing these.

THERAPIST 10: I know. You'd say, "Dad." Yeah.

CLIENT 11: Dad, you . . . [Starts to slump over shaking fists and moaning]

THERAPIST 11: Stay with these feelings, yeah.

CLIENT 12: I am. I'm trying to let them out; I'm not trying to tamp them down.

THERAPIST 12: I know. I know. You're doing great. (Skill 4: Affirming)

CLIENT 13: Dad. . . . How could you have done this to me? It's so wrong. My life is so hard, and it shouldn't be! And you did it. It's your fault. You should have got help and not taken your insecurities out on me. You shouldn't have scared me and belittled me. It had such a big impact on me.

THERAPIST 13: Yeah. That's right. (Skill 4: Affirming)

CLIENT 14: How could you do that? How could you hurt your son so much?

THERAPIST 14: How could you hurt me. Your son. Right. That's right. (Skill 4: Affirming)

CLIENT 15: I don't care how bad your father was . . . it doesn't get you off the hook for what you did.

THERAPIST 15: No, it certainly doesn't. Right. You're doing great. (Skill 4: Affirming) And what does he look like as you tell him this? (Skill 10: Initiating Portrayals)

CLIENT 16: No clue. I have no idea . . . no, maybe I have a clue. The few times I've stood up to him when he is clearly in the wrong, he gets very aggressive. He gets cornered. Because he's not gonna . . . God, I feel better . . . [Leans forward, smiles, looks up and blinks] He's, uh . . .

THERAPIST 16: How do you feel right here? (Skill 11: Privileging Transformance Strivings) You lean forward and smile. (Skill 1: Moment-to-Moment Tracking) Yeah, tell me what you notice inside. (Skill 2: Exploring and Staying With Physical Experience)

CLIENT 17: A sense of partial lightness.

THERAPIST 17: Uh huh. Where do you feel it? (Skill 2: Exploring and Staying With Physical Experience)

CLIENT 18: Yeah, uh, I'm in touch with that feeling.

THERAPIST 18: Yeah. That's great. (Skill 4: Affirming) Where do you notice the partial lightness? (Skill 2: Exploring and Staying With Physical Experience)

CLIENT 19: He would . . . he gets shut down, and he gets . . . like, he would go away in the middle of this; he couldn't hear this.

THERAPIST 19: Yeah. Mhm. So let's . . .

CLIENT 20: I mean, he's not gonna totally break down.

THERAPIST 20: Yeah.

CLIENT 21: So go on. Where do you want to go?

THERAPIST 21: Yeah, so let's stay here: that you feel better. (Skill 11: Privileging Transformance Strivings)

CLIENT 22: Okay.

THERAPIST 22: Because this was a huge, big thing that you did. You said, "I hate doing this," and then you did it, right? (Skill 4: Affirming) And you galvanized yourself to do it, and you really did it. I am so moved that you were so brave to let yourself. (Skill 5: Self-Involving Self-Disclosure) And how do you feel?

CLIENT 23: [Big sigh] Uh. . . . Um . . . it's. . . . How do I feel? Lighter, a bit better. [Another big sigh] . . . You know, very quickly, right now, everything else that's difficult in my life creeps back in. I try to feel better but then like a hole in the sand at the beach it gets washed away.

THERAPIST 23: Uh uh, and you sigh and say, "Yes, I do feel lighter, a bit better." And I feel it too. (Skill 5: Self-Involving Self-Disclosure) You had a moment when you felt better, and then when I said, "You really did it," you galvanized yourself and you did it. It felt to me like you had a moment of, like, "Yeah, I did."

CLIENT 24: Yeah, it was . . . yeah, I did.

THERAPIST 24: Yeah. What was that?

CLIENT 25: It was . . . [Big sigh, slight smile, relaxes and leans back in chair] it was a moment.

THERAPIST 25: Yeah. And you smile and it feels like your body relaxes a bit. (Skill 1: Moment-to-Moment Tracking)

CLIENT 26: Um, right now the waves are so high in my life that the moments don't last long. For that moment, there was a moment of lightness, of . . . okay, relief, lighter . . . you know?

THERAPIST 26: Yeah. And that feeling of lightness, of lighter . . .? (Skill 2: Exploring and Staying With Physical Experience; Skill 11: Privileging Transformance Strivings)

CLIENT 27: Wow, you know I've been saying I really need a day off . . . and I felt for a moment the feeling of a day off, like, one piece of truly feeling a big exhale whew. Oh, wow, I'm here and I'm okay.

THERAPIST 27: Yeah. And what's that like? Again, just to really expand here: "I'm here and I'm okay . . ." (Skill 2: Exploring and Staying With Physical Experience; Skill 11: Privileging Transformance Strivings)

CLIENT 28: It's really good, but at the same time it's really painful. Oh, I really need a lot more. This is weird to say but I almost don't want to feel it because feeling better hurts too.

THERAPIST 28: Yeah, you really need a lot more. Yeah. That's really true. I think you're really right. (Skill 4: Affirming) Yeah. So what's coming up here physically? (Skill 2: Exploring and Staying With Physical Experience)

CLIENT 29: I mean, it's really . . . the last few days have been hard . . . and I do really feel better. A lot better.

THERAPIST 29: Yes, great . . . I really feel like you took a huge, huge step today in actually really changing things. You know? I don't know that you've ever, you know, in your imagination, and here with me, really said what you said about your father, to your father . . . that was a really . . . (Skill 11: Privileging Transformance Strivings)

CLIENT 30: No. No, that's true. I've never spoken up to him before. I've toyed with it, but saying it and . . . I don't feel like I said a hundred percent of it, probably near eighty. And I've never been there any more than ten percent even in my imagination [smiling]. So yeah . . .

THERAPIST 30: So you took a big step, and you had a moment where I said, "You really did it," and you got a smile on your face, you know, just a fleeting one, but I feel like this was a huge step toward freeing yourself from this thing that has been an albatross around your neck—I don't know if I got the metaphors mixed up, a weight, but . . . (Skill 4: Affirming)

CLIENT 31: Yup.

THERAPIST 31: Right. Huge, huge thing. What's it like to really have taken this big step and gone to eighty percent from ten? (Skill 12: Metatherapeutic Processing)

CLIENT 32: I guess I realize I'm thinking of my dad kind of like a cinder block that I'm chained to. And I guess for a few seconds I took it off, and not only did I get to feel what it was like not to have it, but I got to realize that I can take it off . . . which I've never . . . experienced before. Like now I can be rid of him.

THERAPIST 32: Yeah. And what's that like inside? (Skill 2: Exploring and Staying With Physical Experience; Skill 11: Privileging Transformance Strivings)

CLIENT 33: I don't know. That's one I have to chew on a little bit. That's . . . that's some intellectual thinking about that. About what it means—what's happened today, what it means.

THERAPIST 33: What it feels like. Yeah. (Skill 2: Exploring and Staying With Physical Experience)

CLIENT 34: Yeah. So, you're asking me to stay in touch with the few seconds that the hole was unburied and it wasn't full of water?

THERAPIST 34: Yeah, yeah.

CLIENT 35: Okay.

THERAPIST 35: Yeah, and you had a smile on your face. It was fleeting, but it was like, "Yeah, you're right, I galvanized myself and I did it," and I think you felt some pride— I don't wanna presume, but I think you did, and you can see the look on my face full of pride that you did this today. (Skill 5: Self-Involving Self-Disclosure)

CLIENT 36: I did, yeah. I did feel pride. I do feel pride.

THERAPIST 36: Yeah.

CLIENT 37: Yeah.

THERAPIST 37: And you're right that it's fleeting, because you're not used to it. Right?

CLIENT 38: Right, right . . . it's like . . . anything you start doing can be scary at first and you can only do it in short bursts and it hurts at first, but pretty soon it starts to feel good and not so weird and new.

THERAPIST 38: Right . . .

CLIENT 39: And it is scary . . . [Face gets really sad]

THERAPIST 39: Yeah, yeah. I see the sadness. (Skill 1: Moment-to-Moment Tracking) Just stay with this. (Skill 2: Exploring and Staying With Physical Experience)

CLIENT 40: It's, uh . . . [closes eyes, opens them] I don't know. I feel sad, but part of me feels that maybe it's a little . . . I feel like there's a little hope, 'cause it's very true . . . I know how hard it is to go from nothing to something—like meditating. At first you think it's impossible to sit for 5 minutes and then pretty soon you're sitting for 30 minutes and you're like, "Wow I'm doing it!" So maybe it's possible. Maybe I can get there. [Looking really proud: sitting up straight with a slight smile] Maybe.

THERAPIST 40: Yeah, I think so. Definitely. You are already doing it. You are already getting there. (Skill 4: Affirming) And I know personally how hard it is to do this kind of role play. Our histories are different, and I remember the first one I did. So you see I know this difficulty too. (Skill 6: Self-Revealing Self-Disclosure)

CLIENT 41: [Leans forward in chair] You know this too?

THERAPIST 41: I do. I do. How is that to know that about me? (Skill 7: Metaprocessing)

CLIENT 42: Wow. I'm not the only one?

THERAPIST 42: No. No. You're not . . .

CLIENT 43: Wow, of course. I thought like I was the only one and now of course . . . other people have this experience too!

THERAPIST 43: That's right. Other people. Me.

CLIENT 44: [Smiles and looks directly at therapist] You. Thank you for telling me that.

THERAPIST 44: You're welcome. I am glad I did. We're in this together. We really are. (Skill 3: Undoing Aloneness)

CLIENT 45: That's right, and I feel like I just sat down on my meditation cushion—even though that's the wrong image because this was more like taking off my boxing gloves for the first time and seeing my strong hands.

THERAPIST 45: Wow! What a great image! I think you did. I think you did. Good for you! (Skill 4: Affirming) I am so moved by all we did together today. (Skill 5: Self-Involving Self-Disclosure) I'll look forward to seeing you next week.

CLIENT 46: [Smiles broadly] You bet! I'll be here.

THERAPIST 46: [Smiling] Bye.

CLIENT 47: Bye.

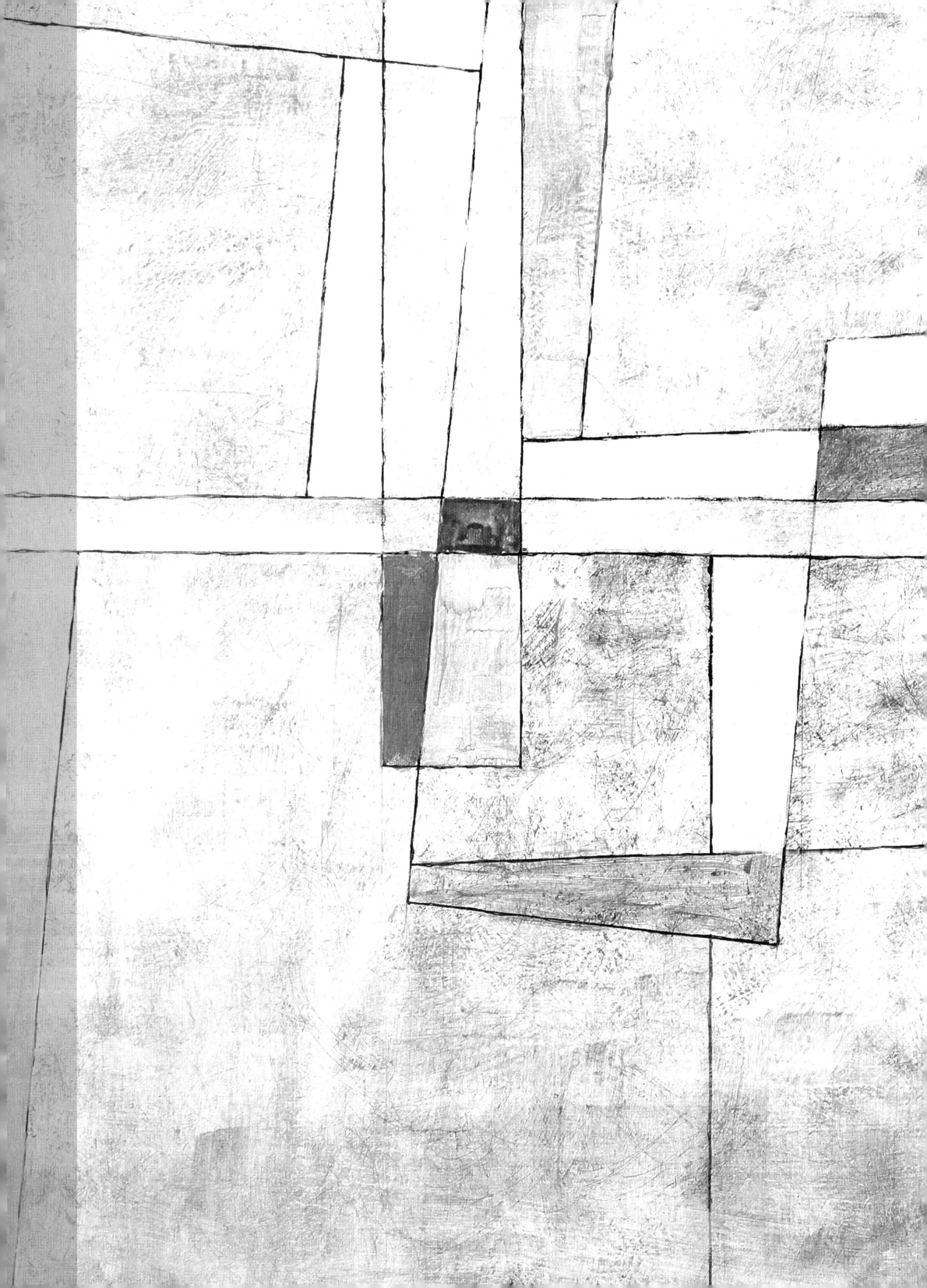

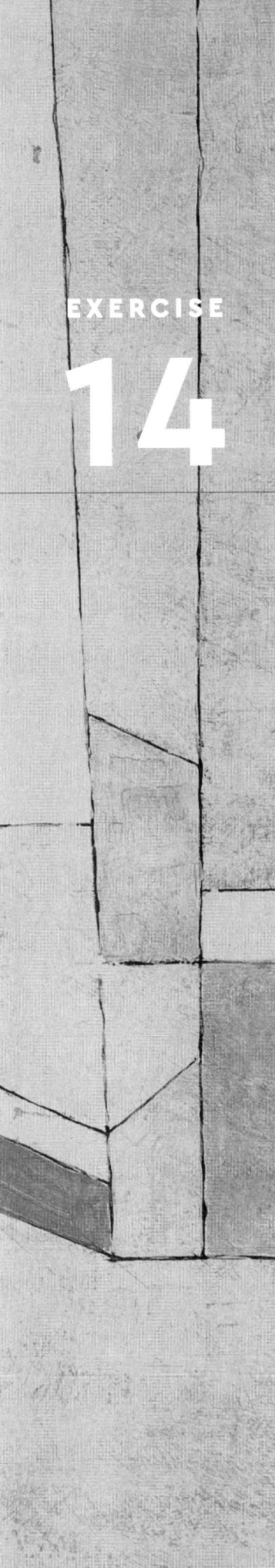

Mock Accelerated Experiential Dynamic Psychotherapy Sessions

In contrast to highly structured and repetitive deliberate practice exercises, a mock accelerated experiential dynamic psychotherapy (AEDP) session is an unstructured and improvised role-play therapy session. Like a jazz rehearsal, mock sessions let you practice the art and science of *appropriate responsiveness* (Hatcher, 2015; Stiles & Horvath, 2017), putting your psychotherapy skills together in a way that is helpful to your mock client. This exercise outlines the procedure for conducting a mock AEDP session. It offers different client profiles you may choose to adopt when role-playing the client.

Mock sessions are an opportunity for trainees to practice the following:

- Using psychotherapy skills responsively.
- Navigating challenging choice-points in therapy.
- Choosing which interventions to use.
- Tracking the arc of a therapy session and the overall big-picture therapy treatment.
- Guiding treatment in the context of the client's preferences.
- Determining realistic goals for therapy in the context of the client's capacities.
- Knowing how to proceed when the therapist is unsure, lost, or confused.
- Recognizing and recovering from therapeutic errors.
- Discovering your personal therapeutic style.
- Building endurance for working with real clients.

Mock Accelerated Experiential Dynamic Psychotherapy Session Overview

For the mock session, **you will perform a role play of an initial therapy session**. As is true with the exercises to build individual skills, the role play involves three people: One trainee role-plays the therapist, another trainee role-plays the client, and a trainer (a professor or a supervisor) observes and provides feedback. This is an open-ended role play, as is commonly done in training. However, this differs in two important ways from the role plays used in more traditional training. First, the therapist will use their

https://doi.org/10.1037/0000439-016

Deliberate Practice in Accelerated Experiential Dynamic Psychotherapy, by N. C. N. Prenn, H. Levenson, A. Vaz, and T. Rousmaniere

hand to indicate how difficult the role play feels. Second, the client will attempt to make the role play easier or harder to ensure the therapist is practicing at the right difficulty level.

Preparation

1. Download the Deliberate Practice Reaction Form and Deliberate Practice Diary Form from the "Resources" tab at https://www.apa.org/pubs/books/deliberate-practice-accelerated-experiential-dynamic-psychotherapy (also available in Appendixes A and B, respectively). Every student will need their own copy of the Deliberate Practice Reaction Form on a separate piece of paper so they can access it quickly.

2. Designate one student to role-play the therapist and one student to role-play the client. The trainer will observe and provide corrective feedback.

Mock Accelerated Experiential Dynamic Psychotherapy Session Procedure

1. The trainees will role-play an initial (first) therapy session. The trainee role-playing the client selects a client profile from the end of this exercise.

2. Before beginning the role play, the therapist raises their hand to their side, at the level of their chair seat (see Figure E14.1). They will use this hand throughout the whole role play to indicate how challenging it feels to them to help the client. Their starting

FIGURE E14.1. Ongoing Difficulty Assessment Through Hand Level

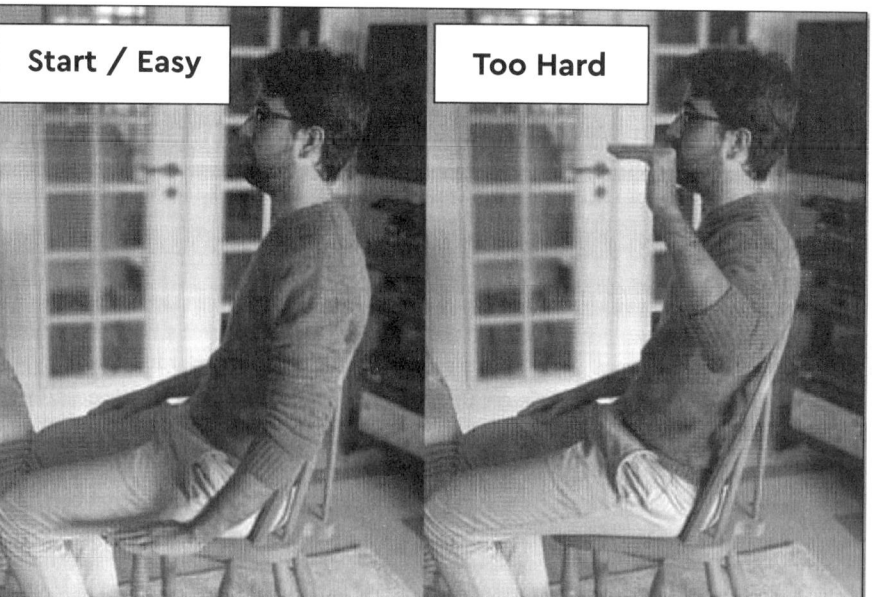

Note. Left: Start of role play. Right: Role play is too difficult. From *Deliberate Practice in Emotion-Focused Therapy* (p. 156), by R. N. Goldman, A. Vaz, and T. Rousmaniere, 2021, American Psychological Association (https://doi.org/10.1037/0000227-000). Copyright 2021 by the American Psychological Association.

hand level (chair seat) indicates that the role play feels easy. By raising their hand, the therapist indicates that the difficulty is rising. If their hand rises above their neck level, it indicates that the role play is too difficult.

3. The therapist begins the role play. The therapist and client should engage in the role play in an improvised manner, as they would engage in a real therapy session. The therapist keeps their hand out at their side throughout this process. (This may feel strange at first!)

4. Whenever the therapist feels that the difficulty of the role play has changed significantly, they should move their hand up if it feels more difficult, down if it feels easier. If the therapist's hand drops below the seat of their chair, the client should make the role play more challenging; if the therapist's hand rises above their neck level, the client should make the role play easier. Instructions for adjusting the difficulty of the role play are described in the "Varying the Level of Challenge" section.

Note to Therapists

Remember to be aware of your vocal quality and nonverbal behavior and movements in doing these role plays. In AEDP, we pay particular attention to how we use our voice (e.g., tone, pacing), facial expressions (e.g., sadness, delight), and nonverbal behavior (e.g., leaning forward or back, hand to heart). For example, you can use your voice quality and pacing to help clients to slow down so they have a better chance to connect with their inner experience. You can also use shifts in vocal quality and nonverbals to express delight and celebratory enthusiasm for the client's progress, imbuing the words with energy, seriousness, and firmness: "You did it! We did it together!"

---

5. The role play continues for at least 15 minutes. The trainer may provide corrective feedback during this process if the therapist gets significantly off-track. However, trainers should exercise restraint and keep feedback as short and tight as possible because this will reduce the therapist's opportunity for experiential training.

6. After the role play is finished, the therapist and client switch roles and begin a new mock session.

7. After both trainees have completed the mock session as a therapist, the trainees and the trainer discuss the experience.

Varying the Level of Challenge

If the therapist indicates that the mock session is too easy, the person enacting the role of the client can use the following modifications to make it more challenging (see also Appendix A):

- The client can improvise with topics that are more evocative or make the therapist uncomfortable, such as displaying no affect or a lot of emotion (see Figure A.2).

- The client can use a distressed voice (upset, angry, sad, sarcastic, etc.) or use expressive face and body movements (make fists, kick a leg out, lean in or back and cross arm, sit immobilized). This gives the trainees more to practice with.

- Blend complex mixtures of opposing feelings (e.g., love and rage).

    If the therapist indicates that the mock session is too hard:

- The client can be guided by Figure A.2 to
    - present topics that are less evocative,
    - present material on any topic but without expressing feelings, or
    - present material concerning the future or the past or events outside therapy.

- The client can ask the questions in a soft voice or with a smile. This softens the emotional stimulus.

- The therapist can take short breaks during the role play.

- The trainer can expand the "feedback phase" by discussing AEDP or psychotherapy theory.

Mock Session Client Profiles

Following are six client profiles for trainees to use during mock sessions, presented in order of difficulty. The choice of client profile may be determined by the trainee playing the therapist, the trainee playing the client, or assigned by the trainer.

The most important aspect of role plays is for trainees to convey the emotional tone indicated by the client profile (e.g., "angry" or "sad"). The demographics of the client (e.g., age, gender) and specific content of the client profiles are not important for practicing the skills. Thus, trainees should adjust the client profile to be most comfortable and easy for the trainee to role-play. For example, a trainee may change the client profile from female to male, from 45 to 22 years old, from transgender to cisgender, and so on.

Beginner Profile: Helping a Receptive Client Process a Breakup With Their Partner

Marco is a 28-year-old software engineer. His boyfriend of 3 years recently broke up with him. It was his first long-term relationship, and now he worries that he will never meet someone he loves as much. He is concerned that he doesn't feel like dating or hooking up. He has been feeling so down that he hasn't been returning his family's texts or phone calls. Instead, he spends his time watching TV and staying up late playing solitary video games. He is depressed, anxious, and, at times, overwhelmingly sad.

- **Symptoms:** Depression and anxiety.

- **Client's goals for therapy:** Marco wants to feel better. He wants to reconnect with friends and family and have hope. He has a small wish that his former partner will recontact him.

- **Attitude toward therapy:** Marco considers his anxiety, sadness, and bouts of crying as signs of weakness. Marco has a best friend who has been helped by therapy and so is willing to come in every week. He has heard from this friend that he should trust the process.

- **Strengths:** Marco has several good friends. Before the breakup, he was an outgoing, thoughtful person who enjoyed his job. He has a long-term perspective that he will get through this loss.

Beginner Profile: Addressing Loneliness and Difficulty Making and Keeping Friends With an Engaged Client

Malia is a 25-year-old working in retail who was recently ghosted by a friend group. She has been having a difficult time keeping in touch with her high school friends and has seen on social media that they are getting together without her. She is wondering if something she is doing has alienated them. She is coming to therapy after a panic attack when she saw a post on social media of a close friend's birthday party to which she was not invited.

- **Symptoms:** Loneliness, anxiety, and panic attack.
- **Client's goals for therapy:** Malia wants to try to figure out if she is doing something to alienate her friends.
- **Attitude toward therapy:** Malia has had a positive experience in therapy for test anxiety when she was in high school. She is hopeful that this therapy will help as well.
- **Strengths:** Malia is emotionally open and motivated to engage in the therapy tasks.

Intermediate Profile: Addressing Anxiety With an Anxious and Preoccupied Client

Connie is a 35-year-old woman who suffers from extreme anxiety stemming from a pre-occupied attachment style and perseverating. Her husband is tired of having to reassure her that he loves her. He gave her an ultimatum to address her anxiety and need for reassurance. Connie is overly attuned to the emotions of others and frequently interprets subtle shifts as signs of rejection and abandonment. She comes by her attachment style honestly. Her parents were unpredictable when she was a child; at times they were loving and attentive and at other times left her abruptly without telling her they were leaving because they wanted to avoid her having a "meltdown." Connie experiences her feelings as overwhelming, and she perseverates on her negative thoughts, doubts, and insecurities. She seeks reassurance to quieten down her worries that she will be left or find herself alone.

- **Symptoms:** Anxiety, an urgent need for reassurance, and insomnia.
- **Client's goals for therapy:** Connie wants someone to talk through the many crises. She thinks of herself as a "relational processor" and so needs to talk.
- **Attitude toward therapy:** Connie is reluctant to be in therapy but is coming because she doesn't want to lose her husband. She has never been in therapy.
- **Strengths:** Underneath her anxiety and preoccupation, Connie wants to connect, and understands intellectually how her need for reassurance pushes people away.

Intermediate Profile: Helping a Client With an Eating Disorder

Dana is a 45-year-old who was encouraged to come to therapy by a friend who noticed that Dana often canceled plans and oscillated between binge eating and not eating. Dana was a latchkey kid and used food to soothe the loneliness and fear from a young age when left home alone. Dana has shame over what feels to them like disgusting behaviors.

- **Symptoms:** Binge eating, restricting, shame, and isolation.
- **Client's goals for therapy:** Dana wants to stop the cycle of binge eating and restricting.
- **Attitude toward therapy:** Dana has never been in therapy before and is ashamed to talk about their "disgusting" behavior around food and needing help.
- **Strengths:** Dana is suffering and is motivated to change.

Advanced Profile: Helping a Highly Intellectual, Defended Client Who Does Not Want to Have Feelings, Anxiety, or Moods

Tyler is a 55-year-old attorney. He is successful at work and considers himself "the rock" of his family. He is coming to therapy because he is wondering if he is having a "midlife crisis." He feels distant from his wife and children and isn't sure he even likes his work. He learned at an early age to depend on himself, which he sees as a strength; he uses his success at work along with joking and self-deprecation to cover over his insecure core. He equates vulnerability with weakness and therefore wants to be "level," as he puts it, without experiencing any emotions at all. He is highly intellectual.

- **Symptoms:** An anxious feeling of dissatisfaction with his life, and insomnia.

- **Client's goals for therapy:** Tyler wants to be "level"—getting back to feeling like his life is going well. He wants to sleep better and not feel so on edge.

- **Attitude toward therapy:** He is distrustful of therapy and afraid that the therapist will want him to cry or "become soft." Down deep he is fearful that he has made a mess of his life and that the work in therapy will confirm it.

- **Strengths:** Tyler is focused and dedicated to anything he puts his mind to. He is resilient and, despite his intellectualization, has some feelings that things are not as they should be.

Advanced Profile: Helping a Client With Posttraumatic Stress Disorder, Suicidal Ideation, and Disorganized Attachment

Isabel is a 22-year-old college student who has lived in the United States for 3 years. She is having problems in her relationships with herself, her boyfriend, and her friends. She experienced criticism, neglect, and physical violence as a child. She is a perfectionist; she is highly critical of herself and others. When she is not living up to her ideals for herself, she gets depressed, self-harms, and experiences suicidal ideation. She oscillates between dismissing the therapist and urgently needing her.

- **Symptoms:** Mood lability, self-harm (cutting), and relationship instability.

- **Client's goals for therapy:** Isabel wants to find stability in herself and her relationships.

- **Attitude toward therapy:** Isabel has been in therapy before but did not think the therapist was smart enough for her. She challenges the therapist and constantly quizzes her about her general knowledge and expertise.

- **Strengths:** Isabel has some insight into her problems and a moderate level of self-awareness.

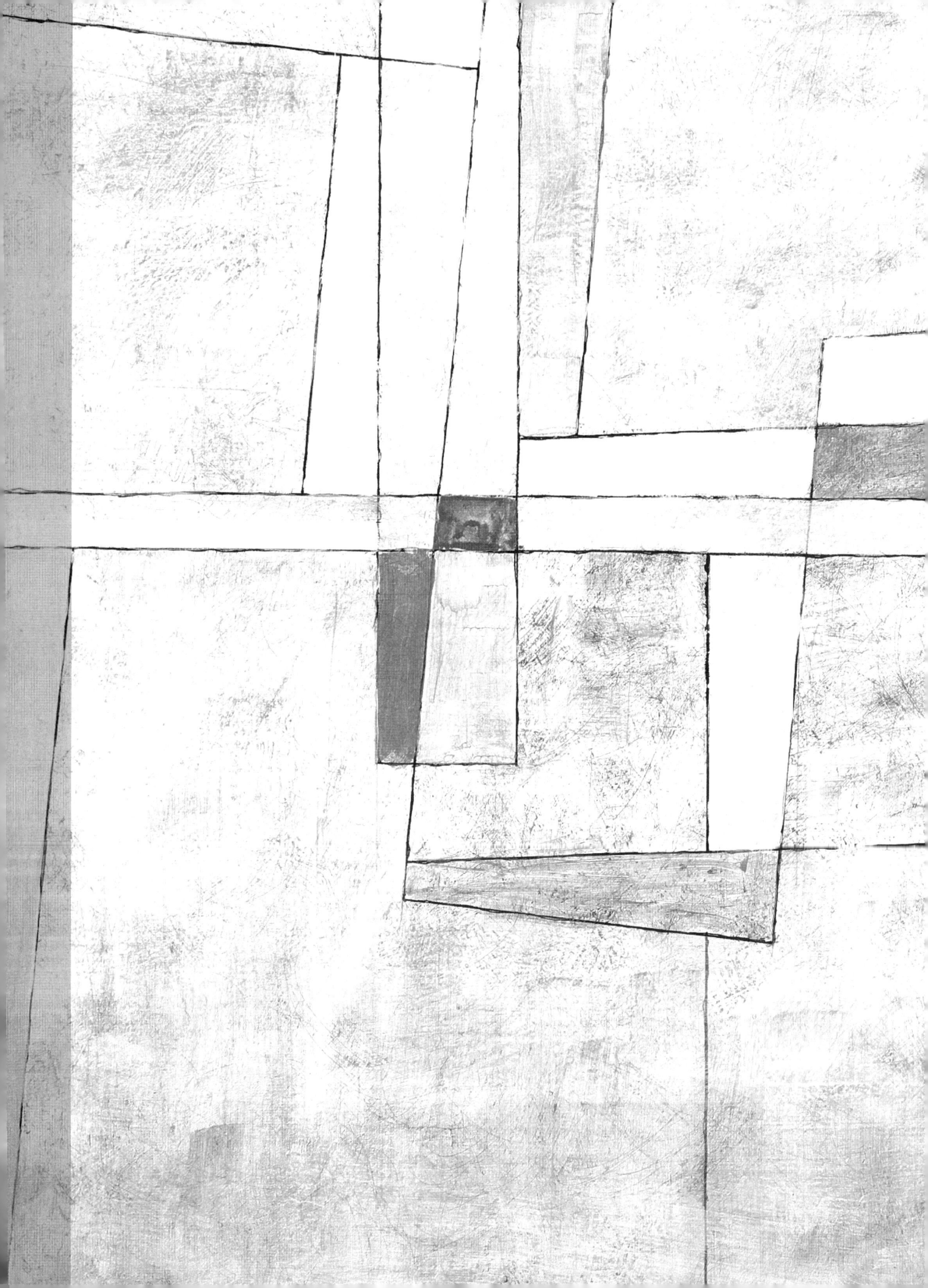

Strategies for Enhancing the Deliberate Practice Exercises

Part III consists of one chapter, Chapter 3, which provides additional advice and instructions for trainers and trainees so that they can reap more benefits from the deliberate practice exercises in Part II. Chapter 3 offers six key points for getting the most out of deliberate practice, guidelines for practicing appropriately responsive treatment, evaluation strategies, methods for ensuring trainee well-being and respecting their privacy, and advice for monitoring the trainer–trainee relationship.

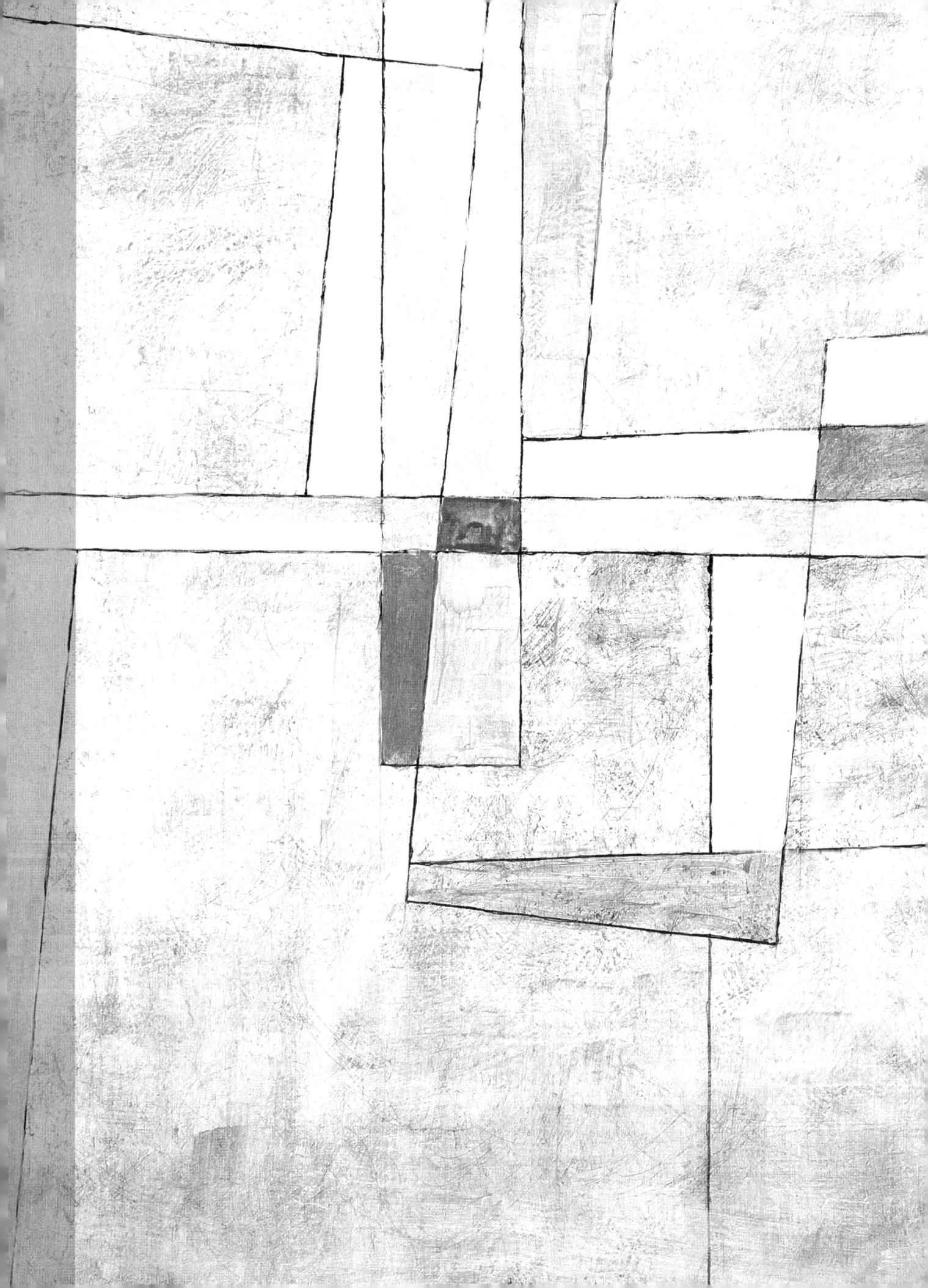

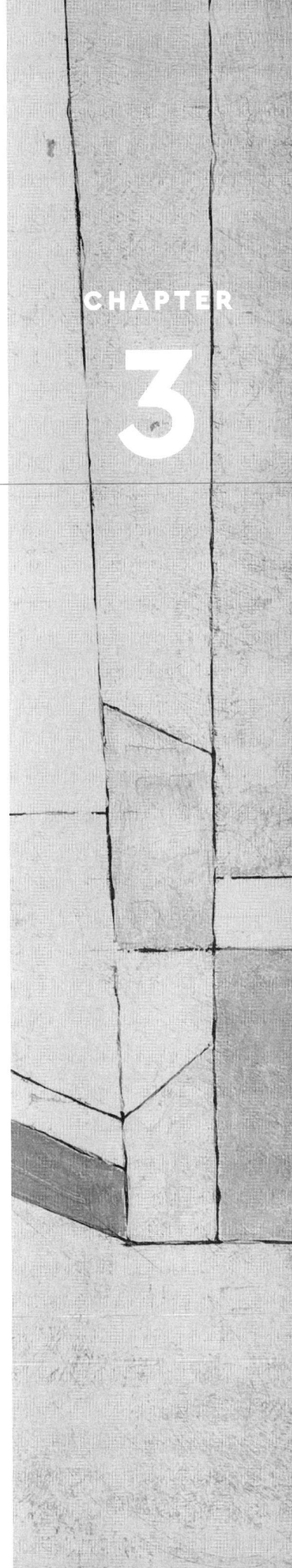

How to Get the Most Out of Deliberate Practice: Additional Guidance for Trainers and Trainees

In Chapter 2 and in the exercises themselves, we have provided instructions for completing these deliberate practice exercises. This chapter provides guidance on big-picture topics that trainers will need to successfully integrate deliberate practice into their training program. This guidance is based on relevant research and the experiences and feedback from trainers at more than a dozen psychotherapy training programs who volunteered to test the deliberate practice exercises in this series. We cover topics including evaluation, getting the most from deliberate practice, trainee well-being, respecting trainee privacy, trainer self-evaluation, responsive treatment, and the trainee–trainer alliance.

Six Key Points for Getting the Most From Deliberate Practice

Following are six key points of advice for trainers and trainees to get the most benefit from the accelerated experiential dynamic psychotherapy (AEDP) deliberate practice exercises. The following advice is gleaned from experiences vetting and practicing deliberate practice exercises, sometimes in different languages, with many trainees, across many countries.

Key Point 1: Create Realistic Emotional Stimuli

A key component of deliberate practice is using stimuli that provoke similar reactions to challenging real-life work settings. For example, pilots train with flight simulators that present mechanical failures and dangerous weather conditions; surgeons practice with surgical simulators that present medical complications with only seconds to respond. Training with challenging stimuli will increase trainees' capacity to perform therapy effectively under stress, for example with clients they find challenging. The stimuli used for AEDP deliberate practice exercises are role plays of challenging client statements in therapy. **It is important that the trainee who is role-playing the client perform the**

https://doi.org/10.1037/0000439-017

Deliberate Practice in Accelerated Experiential Dynamic Psychotherapy, by N. C. N. Prenn, H. Levenson, A. Vaz, and T. Rousmaniere

script with appropriate emotional expression and maintain eye contact with the therapist. For example, if the client statement calls for sad emotion, the trainee should try to express sadness eye-to-eye with the therapist. We offer the suggestions regarding emotional expressiveness:

1. The emotional tone of the role play matters more than the exact words of each script. Trainees role-playing the client should feel free to improvise and change the words if it will help them be more emotionally expressive. Trainees do not need to stick 100% exactly to the script. In fact, to read off the script during the exercise can sound flat and prohibit eye contact. Rather, trainees in the client role should first read the client statement silently to themselves then, when ready, say it in an emotional manner while looking directly at the trainee playing the therapist. This will help the experience feel more real and engaging for the therapist.

2. Trainees whose first language isn't English may particularly benefit from reviewing and changing the words in the client statement script before each role play so that they can find words that feel congruent and facilitate emotional expression.

3. Trainees role-playing the client should try to use tonal and nonverbal expressions of feelings. For example, if a script calls for anger, the trainee can speak with an angry voice and make fists with their hands; if a script calls for shame or guilt, the trainee could hunch over and wince; if a script calls for sadness, the trainee could speak in a soft or quiet voice.

4. If trainees are having persistent difficulties acting believably when following a particular script in the role of client, it may help to first do a "demo round" by reading directly from paper, and then, immediately after, dropping the paper to make eye contact and repeating the same client statement from memory. Some trainees reported this helped them "become available as real clients" and made the role play feel less artificial. Some trainees did three or four "demo rounds" to get fully into their role as a client.

Key Point 2: Customize the Exercises to Fit Your Unique Training Circumstances

Deliberate practice is less about adhering to specific rules than it is about using training principles. Every trainer has their own individual teaching style and every trainee their own learning process. Thus, the exercises in this book are designed to be flexibly customized by trainers across different training contexts within different cultures. Trainees and trainers are encouraged to adjust exercises continually to optimize their practice. The most effective training will occur when deliberate practice exercises are customized to fit the learning needs of each trainee and the culture of each training site. In our experience with numerous trainers and trainees across many countries, we found that everyone spontaneously customized the exercises for their unique training circumstances. No two trainers followed the exact same procedure. For example,

• One supervisor used the exercises with a trainee who found all the client statements to be too hard, including the "beginner" stimuli. This trainee had multiple reactions in the "too hard" category, including nausea, severe shame, and self-doubt. The trainee disclosed to the supervisor that she had experienced extremely harsh learning environments earlier in her life and found the role plays to be highly evocative. To help, the supervisor followed the suggestions offered in Appendix A to make the stimuli progressively easier until the trainee reported feeling a "good challenge" on the Deliberate Practice Reaction Form. Over many weeks of practice, the trainee developed a sense of safety and was able to practice with more difficult client statements. (Note that if the supervisor had proceeded at the too hard difficulty level, the trainee might have complied while hiding her negative reactions, become emotionally flooded and overwhelmed, leading to withdrawal and thus prohibiting her skill development and risking dropout from training.)

- Supervisors of trainees for whom English was not their first language adjusted the client statements to their own primary language.

- One supervisor used the exercises with a trainee who found all the stimuli to be too easy, including the advanced client statements. This supervisor quickly moved to improvising more challenging client statements from scratch by following the instructions in Appendix A on how to make client statements more challenging.

- One supervisor recommended that a trainee use this book as an individual study guide because they were not able to find a suitable partner.

Key Point 3: Discover Your Own Unique Personal Therapeutic Style

Deliberate practice in psychotherapy can be likened to the process of learning to play jazz music. Every jazz musician prides themselves in their skillful improvisations, and the process of "finding your own voice" is a prerequisite for expertise in jazz musicianship. Yet improvisations are not a collection of random notes but the culmination of extensive deliberate practice over time. Indeed, the ability to improvise is built on many hours of dedicated practice of scales, melodies, harmonies, and so on. Much in the same way, psychotherapy trainees are encouraged to experience the scripted interventions in this book not as ends in themselves but as means to promote skill in a systematic fashion. Over time, effective therapeutic creativity can be aided, instead of constrained, by dedicated practice in these therapeutic "melodies." As Philip Glass, the renowned 20th-century American composer, said, "You have to have a place to make the choices from. If you don't have a basis on which to make the choice, then you don't have a style at all, you have a series of accidents" (Glass & Glass, 2012).

Key Point 4: Engage in a Sufficient Amount of Rehearsal

Deliberate practice uses rehearsal to move skills into procedural memory, which helps trainees maintain access to skills even when working with challenging clients. This only works if trainees engage in many repetitions of the exercises. Think of a challenging sport or musical instrument you learned: How many rehearsals would a professional need to feel confident performing a new skill? Psychotherapy is no easier than those other fields!

Key Point 5: Continually Adjust Difficulty

A crucial element of deliberate practice is training at an optimal difficulty level: neither too easy nor too hard. To achieve this, do difficulty assessments and adjustments with the Deliberate Practice Reaction Form in Appendix A. **Do not skip this step!** If trainees don't feel any of the "good challenge" reactions at the bottom of the Deliberate Practice Reaction Form, then the exercise is probably too easy; if they feel any of the "too hard" reactions then the exercise could be too difficult for the trainee to benefit. Advanced trainees and therapists may find all the client statements too easy. If so, they should follow the instructions in Appendix A on making client statements harder to make the role plays sufficiently challenging.

Key Point 6: Putting It All Together With the Practice Transcript and Mock Therapy Sessions

Some trainees may seek greater contextualization of the individual therapy responses associated with each skill, feeling the need to integrate the disparate pieces of their training in a more coherent manner with a simulation that mimics a real therapy session. The annotated transcript in Exercise 13 and the mock therapy sessions in Exercise 14 give trainees this opportunity, allowing them to practice delivering different responses sequentially in a more realistic therapeutic encounter.

Responsive Treatment

The exercises in this book are designed not only to help trainees acquire specific skills of AEDP but to use them in ways that are responsive to each individual client. Across the psychotherapy literature, this stance has been referred to as *appropriate responsiveness*, wherein the therapists exercise flexible judgment, based in their perception of the client's emotional state, needs, and goals, and integrates techniques and other interpersonal skills in pursuit of optimal client outcomes (Hatcher, 2015; Stiles, Honos-Webb & Surko, 1998). The effective therapist is responsive to the emerging context. As Stiles and Horvath (2017) argued, therapists are effective because they are appropriately responsive. Doing the "right thing" may be different each time and means providing each client with an individually tailored response.

Appropriate responsiveness counters a misconception that deliberate practice rehearsal is designed to promote robotic repetition of therapy techniques. Psychotherapy researchers have shown that overadherence to a particular model while neglecting client preferences reduces therapy effectiveness (e.g., Castonguay et al., 1996; Henry et al., 1993; Owen & Hilsenroth, 2014). Therapist flexibility, on the other hand, has been shown to improve outcomes (e.g., Bugatti & Boswell, 2016; Kendall & Beidas, 2007; Kendall & Frank, 2018). It is important, therefore, that trainees practice their newly learned skills in a manner that is flexible and responsive to the unique needs of a diverse range of clients (Hatcher, 2015; Hill & Knox, 2013). It is thus of paramount importance for trainees to develop the necessary perceptual skills to be able to attune to what the client is experiencing in the moment and form their response based on the client moment-by-moment context (Greenberg & Goldman, 1988).

Supervisors must help supervisees attune themselves specifically to the unique and specific needs of the clients during sessions.

> Being exquisitely attuned to the vicissitudes of client engagement, that is, what we call moment-to-moment tracking, characterizes and underlies AEDP therapy and supervision and is something that we explicitly teach. Also AEDP supervision and training's reliance on the use of video further allows accurate attunement to become an achievable reality and not a merely wished for, but unreachable, competency. (Prenn & Fosha, 2017, pp. 147–148)

AEDP supervision uses the viewing of video recordings of the trainee's actual therapy sessions rather than trusting self-report alone. "The video recording provides . . . feedback to the therapist—feedback that is decoded, interpreted, and elaborated in the supervision session; there, the feedback is held and supported within the cocreated safety of AEDP supervision" (Prenn & Fosha, 2017, p. 145). In their 2017 book, Prenn and Fosha pointed out that the supervisee's preparing for supervision by watching a video of their session and looking for places that represent clinical challenges to bring to supervision for feedback reflect the essence of deliberate practice.

By enacting responsiveness with the supervisee, the supervisor can demonstrate its value and make it more explicit. In these ways, attention can be given to the larger picture of appropriate responsiveness. Here the trainee and supervisor can work together to help the trainee master not just the techniques, but how the therapist can use their judgment to put the techniques together to foster positive change. Helping trainees keep this overarching goal in mind while reviewing the therapy process is a valuable feature of supervision that is difficult to obtain otherwise (Hatcher, 2015).

It is also important that deliberate practice occurs within a context of wider AEDP learning. As noted in Chapter 1, training should be combined with supervision of actual therapy recordings, theoretical learning, observation of competent AEDP psychotherapists, as well as personal therapeutic work. When the trainer or trainee determines that the trainee is having difficulty acquiring AEDP skills, it is important to assess carefully what is missing or needed. Assessment should then lead to the appropriate remedy, as the trainer and trainee collaboratively determine what is needed.

Being Mindful of Trainee Well-Being

Although negative effects that some clients experience in psychotherapy have been well documented (Barlow, 2010), negative effects of training and supervision on trainees has received less attention (Ellis et al., 2014). AEDP has a strong tradition of creating and sustaining safety in training and supervision, much as it does in working with clients. The supervisory and training relationship is built on warmth, empathy, and a validating bond. The supervisor or trainer helps the trainee have transformational learning experiences by fostering a sense of authenticity and collaboration in the safety of the dyadic supervisory relationship.

To support strong self-efficacy, trainers must ensure that trainees are practicing at a correct difficulty level. The exercises in this book feature guidance for frequently assessing and adjusting the difficulty level so that trainees can rehearse at a level that precisely targets their personal skill threshold. Trainers and supervisors must be mindful to provide an appropriate challenge. One risk to trainees that is particularly pertinent to this book occurs when using role plays that are too difficult. The Deliberate Practice Reaction Form in Appendix A is provided to help trainers ensure that role plays are done at an appropriate challenge level. Trainers or trainees may be tempted to skip the difficulty assessments and adjustments, out of their motivation to focus on rehearsal to make fast progress and quickly acquire skills. But across all our test sites, we found that skipping the difficulty assessments and adjustments caused more problems and hindered skill acquisition more than any other error. Thus, trainers are advised to remember that **one of their most important responsibilities is to remind trainees to do the difficulty assessments and adjustments**.

Additionally, the Deliberate Practice Reaction Form serves a dual purpose of helping trainees develop the important skills of self-monitoring and self-awareness (Bennett-Levy, 2019). This will help trainees adopt a positive and empowered stance regarding their own self-care and should facilitate career-long professional development.

Respecting Trainee Privacy

The deliberate practice exercises in this book may stir up complex or uncomfortable personal reactions within trainees, including, for example, memories of past trauma. Exploring psychological and emotional reactions may make some trainees feel vulnerable. Therapists of every career stage, from trainees to seasoned therapists with decades of experience, commonly experience shame, embarrassment, and self-doubt in this process. Although these experiences can be valuable for building trainees' self-awareness, it is important that training remain focused on professional skill development and not blur into personal therapy (e.g., Ellis et al., 2014). Therefore, one trainer role is to remind trainees to maintain appropriate boundaries.

Trainees must have the final say about what to disclose or not disclose to their trainer. Trainees should keep in mind that the goal is for the trainee to expand their own self-awareness and psychological capacity to stay active and helpful while experiencing uncomfortable reactions. The trainer does not need to know the specific details about the trainee's inner world for this to happen.

Trainees should be instructed to share only personal information that they feel comfortable sharing. The Deliberate Practice Reaction Form and difficulty assessment process is designed to help trainees build their self-awareness while retaining control over their privacy. Trainees can be reminded that the goal is for them to learn about their own inner world. They do not necessarily have to share that information with trainers or peers (Bennett-Levy & Finlay-Jones, 2018). Likewise, trainees should be instructed to respect the confidentiality of their peers.

Trainer Self-Evaluation

The exercises in this book were tested at a wide range of training sites around the world, including graduate courses, practicum sites, and private practice offices. Although trainers reported that the exercises were highly effective for training, some also said that they felt disoriented by how different deliberate practice feels compared with their traditional methods of clinical education. Many felt comfortable evaluating their trainees' performance but were less sure about their own performance as trainers.

The most common concern we heard from trainers was, "My trainees are doing great, but I'm not sure if I am doing this correctly!" To address this concern, we recommend trainers perform periodic self-evaluations along the following five criteria:

1. Observe trainees' work performance.
2. Provide continual corrective feedback.
3. Ensure rehearsal of specific skills is just beyond the trainees' current ability.
4. Ensure that the trainee is practicing at the right difficulty level (neither too easy nor too challenging).
5. Continuously assess trainee performance with real clients.

Criterion 1: Observe Trainees' Work Performance

Determining how well we are doing as trainers means first having valid information about how well trainees are responding to training. This requires that we directly observe trainees practicing skills to provide corrective feedback and evaluation. One risk of deliberate practice is that trainees gain competence in performing therapy skills in role plays, but those skills do not transfer to trainees' work with real clients. Thus, trainers will ideally also have the opportunity to observe samples of trainees' work with real clients, either live or via recorded video. Supervisors and consultants rely heavily—and, too often, exclusively—on supervisees' and consultees' narrative accounts of their work with clients (Goodyear & Nelson, 1997). Haggerty and Hilsenroth (2011) described this challenge:

> Suppose a loved one has to undergo surgery and you need to choose between two surgeons, one of whom has never been directly observed by an experienced surgeon while performing any surgery. He or she would perform the surgery and return to his or her attending physician and try to recall, sometimes incompletely or inaccurately, the intricate steps of the surgery they just performed. It is hard to imagine that anyone, given a choice, would prefer this over a professional who has been routinely observed in the practice of their craft. (p. 193)

Criterion 2: Provide Continual Corrective Feedback

Trainees need corrective feedback to learn what they are doing well, doing poorly, and how to improve their skills. Feedback should be as specific and incremental as possible. The following are examples of specific feedback: "Your voice sounds rushed. Try slowing down by pausing for a few seconds between your statements to the client" and "That's excellent how you are making eye contact with the client." Examples of vague and nonspecific feedback are "Try to build better rapport with the client" and "Try to be more open to the client's feelings."

Criterion 3: Specific Skill Rehearsal Just Beyond the Trainees' Current Ability (Zone of Proximal Development)

Deliberate practice emphasizes skill acquisition via behavioral rehearsal. Trainers should endeavor not to get caught up in client conceptualization at the expense of focusing on skills. For many trainers, this requires significant discipline and self-restraint. It is simply more enjoyable to talk about psychotherapy theory (e.g., case conceptualization, treatment planning, nuances of psychotherapy models, similar cases the supervisor has had) than watch trainees rehearse skills. Trainees have many questions, and supervisors have an abundance of experience; the allotted supervision time can easily be filled sharing knowledge. The supervisor gets to sound smart, while the trainee doesn't have to struggle with acquiring skills at their learning edge. Although answering questions is important, trainees' intellectual knowledge about psychotherapy can quickly surpass their procedural ability to perform psychotherapy, particularly with clients they find challenging. Here's a simple rule of thumb: The trainer provides the knowledge, but the behavioral rehearsal provides the skill (Rousmaniere, 2019).

Criterion 4: Practice at the Right Difficulty Level (Neither Too Easy nor Too Challenging)

Deliberate practice involves *optimal strain*: practicing skills just beyond the trainee's current skill threshold so that they can learn incrementally without becoming overwhelmed (Ericsson, 2006).

Trainers should use difficulty assessments and adjustments throughout deliberate practice to ensure that trainees are practicing at the right difficulty level. Note that some trainees are surprised by their unpleasant reactions to exercises (e.g., dissociation, nausea, blanking out), and may be tempted to "push through" exercises that are too hard. This can happen out of fear of failing a course, fear of being judged as incompetent, or negative self-impressions by the trainee (e.g., "This shouldn't be so hard"). Trainers should normalize the fact that there will be wide variation in perceived difficulty of the exercises and encourage trainees to respect their own personal training process.

Criterion 5: Continuously Assess Trainee Performance With Real Clients

The goal of deliberately practicing psychotherapy skills is to improve trainees' effectiveness at helping real clients. One of the risks in deliberate practice training is that the benefits will not generalize: Trainees' acquired competence in specific skills may not translate into work with real clients. Thus, it is important that trainers assess the impact of deliberate practice on trainees' work with real clients. Ideally, this is done through triangulation of multiple data points:

- Client data (verbal self-report and routine outcome monitoring data)
- Supervisor's report
- Trainee's self-report

If the trainee's effectiveness with real clients is not improving after deliberate practice, the trainer should do a careful assessment of the difficulty. If the supervisor or trainer feels it is a skill acquisition issues, they may want to consider adjusting the deliberate practice routine to better suit the trainee's learning needs or style.

Therapists have traditionally been evaluated from a lens of *process accountability* (Markman & Tetlock, 2000; see also Goodyear, 2015), which focuses on demonstrating specific behaviors (e.g., fidelity to a treatment model) without regard to the impact on clients. We propose that clinical effectiveness is better assessed through a lens tightly focused on client outcomes and that learning objectives shift from performing behaviors that experts have decided are effective (i.e., the competence model) to highly individualized behavioral goals tailored to each trainee's zone of proximal development and performance feedback. This model of assessment has been termed *outcome accountability* (Goodyear, 2015), which focuses on client changes, rather than therapist competence, independent of how the therapist might be performing expected tasks.

Guidance for Trainees

The central theme of this book has been that skill rehearsal is not automatically helpful. Deliberate practice must be done well for trainees to benefit (Ericsson & Pool, 2016). In this chapter and in the exercises, we offer guidance for effective deliberate practice. We would also like to provide additional advice specifically for trainees. That advice is drawn from what we have learned at our volunteer deliberate practice test sites around the world. We cover how to discover your own training process, active effort, playfulness, and taking breaks during deliberate practice; your right to control your self-disclosure to trainers; monitoring training results; monitoring complex reactions toward the trainer; and your own personal therapy.

Individualized Accelerated Experiential Dynamic Psychotherapy Training: Finding Your Zone of Proximal Development

Deliberate practice works best when training targets each trainee's personal skill thresholds. Also termed the *zone of proximal development*, a term first coined by Vygotsky in reference to developmental learning theory (Zaretskii, 2009), this is the area just beyond the trainee's current ability but that is possible to reach with the assistance of a teacher or coach (Wass & Golding, 2014). **If a deliberate practice exercise is either too easy or too hard, the trainee will not benefit.** To maximize training productivity, elite performers follow a "challenging but not overwhelming" principle: Tasks that are too far beyond their capacity will prove ineffective and even harmful, and it is equally true that mindlessly repeating what they already can do confidently will prove fruitless. Because of this, deliberate practice requires ongoing assessment of the trainee's current skill and concurrent difficulty adjustment to target a "good enough" challenge consistently. Thus, if you are practicing Exercise 8, Working With Anxiety, and it just feels too difficult, consider moving back to a more comfortable skill such as Exercise 4, Affirming, that you may feel you have already mastered.

Active Effort

It is important for trainees to maintain an active and sustained effort while doing the deliberate practice exercises in this book. Deliberate practice really helps when trainees push themselves up to and past their current ability. This is best achieved when trainees take ownership of their own practice by guiding their training partners to adjust role plays to be as high on the difficulty scale as possible without hurting themselves. This will look different for every trainee. Although it can feel uncomfortable or even frightening, this is the zone of proximal development where the most gains can be made. Simply reading and repeating the written scripts will provide little or no benefit. Trainees are advised to remember that their effort from training should lead to more confidence and comfort in session with real clients.

Stay the Course: Effort Versus Flow

Deliberate practice only works if trainees push themselves hard enough to break out of their old patterns of performance, which then permits growth of new skills (Ericsson & Pool, 2016). Because deliberate practice constantly focuses on the current edge of one's performance capacity, it is inevitably a straining endeavor. Indeed, professionals are unlikely to make lasting performance improvements unless there is sufficient engagement in tasks that are just at the edge of one's current capacity (Ericsson, 2003, 2006). From athletics or fitness training, many of us are familiar with this process of being pushed out of our comfort zones followed by adaptation. The same process applies to our mental and emotional abilities.

Many trainees might be surprised to discover that deliberate practice for AEDP feels harder than psychotherapy with a real client. This may be because when working with a real client, a therapist can get into a state of *flow* (Csikszentmihalyi, 1997), where work feels effortless. For example, a trainee at one of our test sites, did just fine with most of the beginner exercises, but when it came to tracking the nonverbal actions of the client (Exercise 1), something at which she did not feel proficient, she felt exhausted doing it. In such cases, it may be wise for trainees to move to offering response formats with which they are more familiar and feel more proficient, and try those for a short time, in part to increase a sense of confidence and mastery.

Discover Your Own Training Process

The effectiveness of deliberate practice is directly related to the effort and ownership trainees exert while doing the exercises. Trainers can provide guidance, but it is important for trainees to learn about their own idiosyncratic training processes over time. This will let them become masters of their own training and prepare for a career-long process of professional development. The following are a few examples of personal training processes trainees discovered while engaging in deliberate practice:

- One trainee noticed that she was good at persisting while an exercise is challenging but also that she requires more rehearsal than other trainees to feel comfortable with a new skill. This trainee focused on developing patience with her own pace of progress.

- One trainee noticed that he could acquire new skills rather quickly, with only a few repetitions. However, he also noticed that his reactions to evocative client statements could jump quickly and unpredictably from the "good challenge" to "too hard" categories, so he needed to attend carefully to the reactions listed in the Deliberate Practice Reaction Form.

- One trainee described herself as "perfectionistic" and felt a strong urge to "push through" an exercise even when she had anxiety reactions in the "too hard" category, such as nausea and dissociation. This caused the trainee not to benefit from the exercises and risk feeling demoralized. This trainee focused on going slower, developing self-compassion regarding her anxiety reactions, and asking her training partners to make role plays less challenging.

Trainees are encouraged to reflect deeply on their own experiences using the exercises to learn the most about themselves and their personal learning processes.

Playfulness and Taking Breaks

Psychotherapy is serious work that often involves painful feelings. However, practicing psychotherapy can be playful and fun (Scott Miller, personal communication, 2017). Trainees should remember that one of the main goals of deliberate practice is to experiment with different approaches and styles of therapy. If deliberate practice ever feels rote, boring, or routine, it probably isn't going to help advance trainees' skill. In this case, trainees should try to liven it up. A good way to do this is to introduce an atmosphere of playfulness. For example, trainees can try the following:

- Use different vocal tones, speech pacing, body gestures, or other languages. This can expand trainees' communication range.

- Practice while closing one's eyes or turning off the sound while watching a video. This can increase awareness coming from other sensory input.

- Practice while standing up or walking around outside. This can help trainees gain new perspectives on the process of therapy.

The supervisor can also ask trainees if they would like to take a 5- to 10-minute break between questions, particularly if the trainees are dealing with difficult emotions and are feeling stressed.

Additional Deliberate Practice Opportunities

This book focuses on deliberate practice methods that involve active, live engagement between trainees and a supervisor. However, deliberate practice can extend beyond these focused training sessions. This book can be used for individual study and homework. For example, a trainee might read the client statements and practice their responses independently between sessions. In such cases, it is important for the trainee to say their therapist responses aloud, rather than rehearse silently in their head. Alternatively, two trainees can practice as a pair, without the supervisor. Although the absence of a supervisor limits one source of feedback, the peer trainee who is playing the client can serve this role. Also, we have had trainees who have used videos of their client sessions as stimuli, stopping the video at a place of clinical challenge and practicing responses said aloud to the clients on the screen. Doing this for a skill deficit that had been previously identified by a supervisor is particularly beneficial. Using video, as in these examples, is an excellent way to approximate the reality of a clinical session.

To optimize the quality of the deliberate practice when conducted independently or without a supervisor, we have developed a Deliberate Practice Diary Form that can be found in Appendix B or downloaded from https://www.apa.org/pubs/books/deliberate-practice-accelerated-experiential-dynamic-psythotherapy (see the "Resources" tab). This form provides a template for the trainee to record their experience of the deliberate practice activity, and, ideally, it will aid in the consolidation of learning. This form can be used as part of the evaluation process with the supervisor but is not necessarily intended for that purpose, and trainees are certainly welcome to bring their experience with the independent practice into the next meeting with the supervisor.

Monitoring Training Results

While trainers will evaluate trainees using a competency-focused model, trainees are also encouraged to take ownership of their own training process and look for results of deliberate practice themselves. Trainees should experience the results of deliberate practice within a few training sessions. A lack of results can be demoralizing for trainees and result in their applying less effort and focus in deliberate practice. Trainees who are not seeing results should openly discuss this problem with their trainer and experiment with adjusting their deliberate practice process. Results can include client outcomes and improving the trainee's own work as a therapist, their personal development, and their overall training.

Client Outcomes

The most important result of deliberate practice is an improvement in trainees' client outcomes. This can be assessed via routine outcome measurement (Lambert, 2010; Miller et al., 2018), qualitative data (McLeod, 2017), and informal discussions with clients. However, trainees should note that an improvement in client outcome due to deliberate practice can sometimes be challenging to achieve quickly, given that the largest amount of variance in client outcome is due to client variables (Bohart & Wade, 2013). For example, a client with severe chronic symptoms may not respond quickly to any treatment, regardless of how effectively a trainee practices. For some clients, an increase in patience and self-compassion regarding their symptoms may be a sign of progress, rather than an immediate decrease in symptoms. Thus, trainees are advised to keep their expectations for client change realistic in the context of their client's symptoms, history, and presentation. It is important that trainees do not try to force their clients to improve in therapy so that the trainee feels like they are making progress in their training (Rousmaniere, 2016).

Trainee's Work as a Therapist

One important result of deliberate practice is change within the trainee regarding their work with clients. For example, trainees at test sites reported feeling more comfortable sitting with evocative clients, more confident addressing uncomfortable topics in therapy, and more responsive to a broader range of clients.

Trainee's Personal Development

Another important result of deliberate practice is personal growth within the trainee. For example, trainees at test sites reported becoming more in touch with their own feelings, increased self-compassion, and enhanced motivation to work with a broader range of clients.

Trainee's Training Process

Another valuable result of deliberate practice is improvement in the trainees' training process. For example, trainees at test sites reported becoming more aware of their personal training style, preferences, strengths, and challenges. Over time, trainees should grow to feel more ownership of their training process. It is also recommended that training to be a psychotherapist is a complex process that occurs over many years. Experienced, expert therapists still report continuing to grow well beyond their graduate school years (Orlinsky & Ronnestad, 2005). I (H. L.) have been doing therapy for almost 50 years. And yet it is a rare week when I don't learn something new or am confronted with a situation where I come up against a clinical challenge or skill deficit. Remember, be easy on yourself!

The Trainee–Trainer Alliance: Monitoring Complex Reactions Toward the Trainer

Trainees who engage in hard deliberate practice often report experiencing complex feelings toward their trainer. For example, one trainee said, "I know this is helping, but I also don't look forward to it!" Another trainee reported feeling both appreciation and frustration towards her trainer simultaneously. Trainees are advised to remember intensive training they have done in other fields, such as athletics or music. When a coach pushes a trainee to the edge of their ability, it is common for trainees to have complex reactions towards them.

This does not necessarily mean that the trainer is doing anything wrong. In fact, intensive training inevitably stirs up reactions toward the trainer, such as frustration, annoyance, disappointment, or anger that coexist with the appreciations they feel. In fact, if trainees do not experience complex reactions, it is worth considering if the deliberate practice is sufficiently challenging. But what we asserted earlier about rights to privacy apply here as well. Because professional mental health training is hierarchical and evaluative, trainers should not require or even expect trainees to share complex reactions they may be experiencing toward them. Trainers should stay open to their sharing, but the choice always remains with the trainee.

Trainee's Own Therapy

When engaging in deliberate practice, many trainees discover aspects of their inner world that may benefit from attending their own psychotherapy. For example, one trainee discovered that her clients' anger stirred up her own painful memories of abuse, another trainee found himself disassociating while practicing empathy skills, and another trainee experienced overwhelming shame and self-judgment when they couldn't master skills after just a few repetitions.

While these discoveries were unnerving at first, they ultimately were beneficial, as they motivated the trainees to seek out their own therapy. Many therapists attend their own therapy. In fact, Norcross and Guy (2005) found in their review of 17 studies that about 75% of the more than 8,000 therapist participants have attended their own therapy. Orlinsky and Ronnestad (2005) found that more than 90% of therapists who attended their own therapy reported it as helpful.

QUESTIONS FOR TRAINEES

1. Are you balancing the effort to improve your skills with patience and self-compassion for your learning process?

2. Are you attending to feelings of shame or self-judgment that are arising from your training?

3. Are you being mindful of your personal boundaries and also respecting any complex feelings you may have towards your trainers?

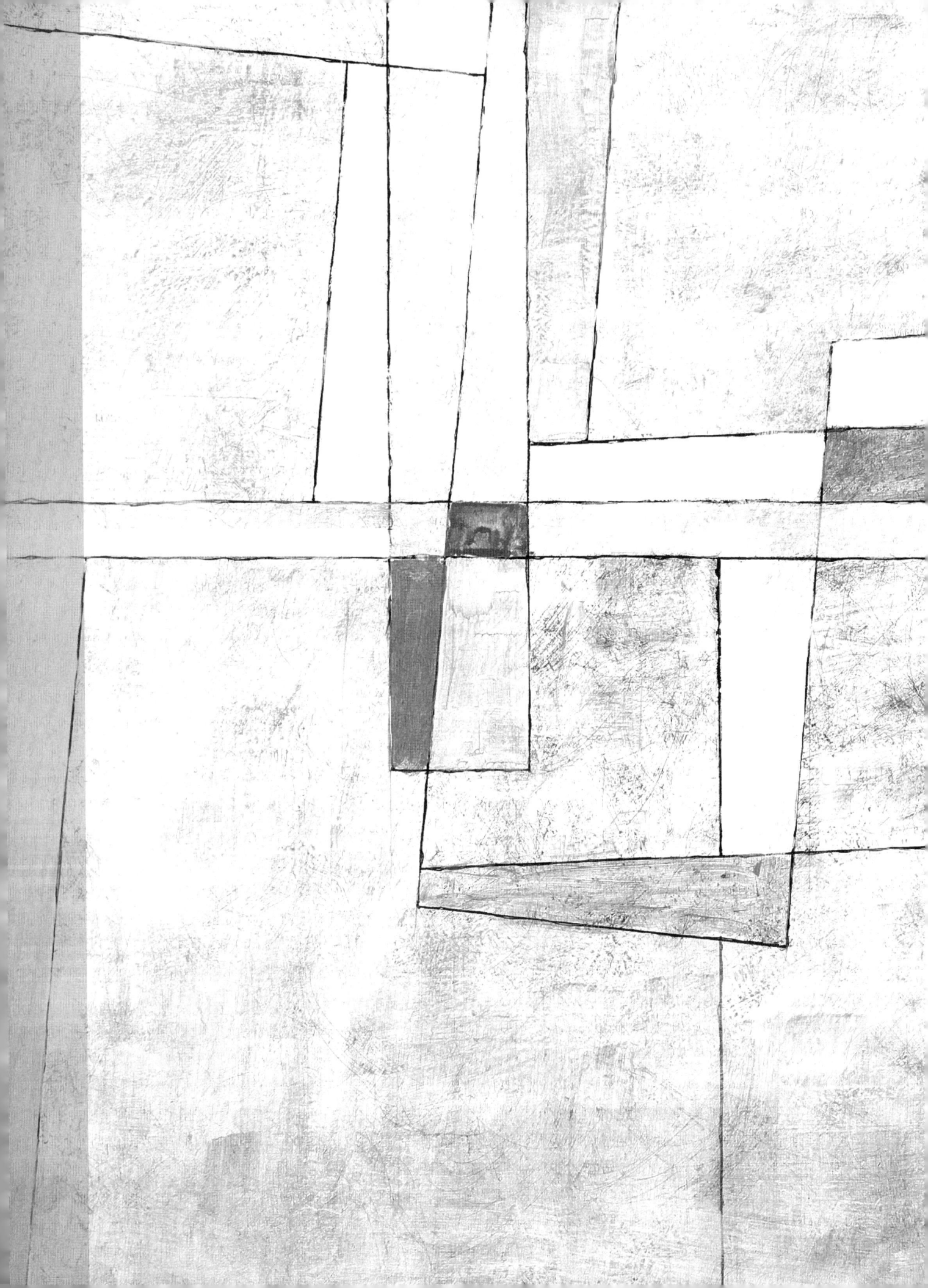

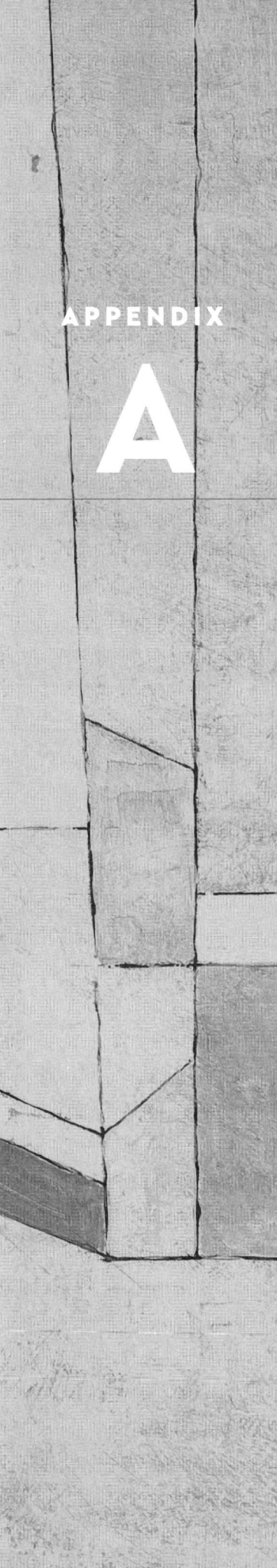

Difficulty Assessments and Adjustments

Deliberate practice works best if the exercises are performed at a good challenge that is neither too hard nor too easy. To ensure that they are practicing at the correct difficulty, trainees should do a difficulty assessment and adjustment after each level of client statement is completed (beginner, intermediate, and advanced). To do this, use the following instructions and the Deliberate Practice Reaction Form (Figure A.1), which is also available in the "Resources" tab at https://www.apa.org/pubs/books/deliberate-practice-accelerated-experiential-dynamic-psychotherapy. **Do not skip this process!**

How to Assess Difficulty

The therapist completes the reaction form (Figure A.1). If they

- rate the difficulty of the exercise above an 8 or had any of the reactions in the "Too Hard" column, follow the instructions to make the exercise easier;

- rate the difficulty of the exercise below a 4 or didn't have any of the reactions in the "Good Challenge" column, proceed to the next level of harder client statements or follow the instructions to make exercise harder; or

- rate the difficulty of the exercise between 4 and 8 and have at least one reaction in the "Good Challenge" column, do not proceed to the harder client statements but rather repeat the same level.

Making Client Statements Easier

If the therapist ever rates the difficulty of the exercise above an 8 or has any of the reactions in the "Too Hard" column, use the next-level easier client statements (e.g., if you were using advanced client statements, switch to intermediate). But if you were already using beginner client statements, use the following methods to make the client statements even easier:

- The person playing the client can use the same beginner client statements but this time in a softer, calmer voice and with a smile. This softens the emotional tone.

FIGURE A.1. Deliberate Practice Reaction Form

Question 1: How challenging was it to fulfill the skill criteria for this exercise?

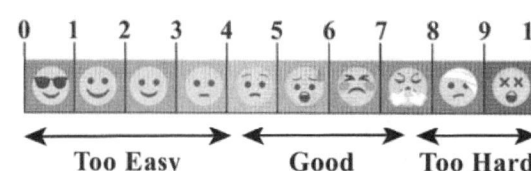

Question 2: Did you have any reactions in "good challenge" or "too hard" categories? (yes/no)					
Good Challenge			**Too Hard**		
Emotions and Thoughts	Body Reactions	Urges	Emotions and Thoughts	Body Reactions	Urges
Manageable shame, self-judgment, irritation, anger, sadness, etc.	Body tension, sighs, shallow breathing, increased heart rate, warmth, dry mouth	Looking away, withdrawing, changing focus	Severe or overwhelming shame, self-judgment, rage, grief, guilt, etc.	Migraines, dizziness, foggy thinking, diarrhea, disassociation, numbness, blanking out, nausea, etc.	Shutting down, giving up

Too Easy ⬇ Proceed to next difficulty level	**Good Challenge** ⬇ Repeat the same difficulty level	**Too Hard** ⬇ Go back to previous difficulty level

Note. From *Deliberate Practice in Emotion-Focused Therapy* (p. 180), by R. N. Goldman, A. Vaz, and T. Rousmaniere, 2021, American Psychological Association (https://doi.org/10.1037/0000227-000). Copyright 2021 by the American Psychological Association.

- The client can improvise with topics that are less evocative or make the therapist more comfortable, such as talking about topics without expressing feelings, the future or past (avoiding the here-and-now), or any topic outside therapy (see Figure A.2).

- The therapist can take a short break (5–10 minutes) between questions.

- The trainer can expand the "feedback phase" by discussing accelerated experiential dynamic psychotherapy or psychotherapy theory and research. This should shift the trainees' focus toward more detached or intellectual topics and reduce the emotional intensity.

Making Client Statements Harder

If the therapist rates the difficulty of the exercise below a 4 or didn't have any of the reactions in the "Good Challenge" column, proceed to next-level harder client statements. If you were already using the advanced client statements, the client should make the exercise even harder, using the following guidelines:

FIGURE A.2. How to Make Client Statements Easier or Harder in Role Plays

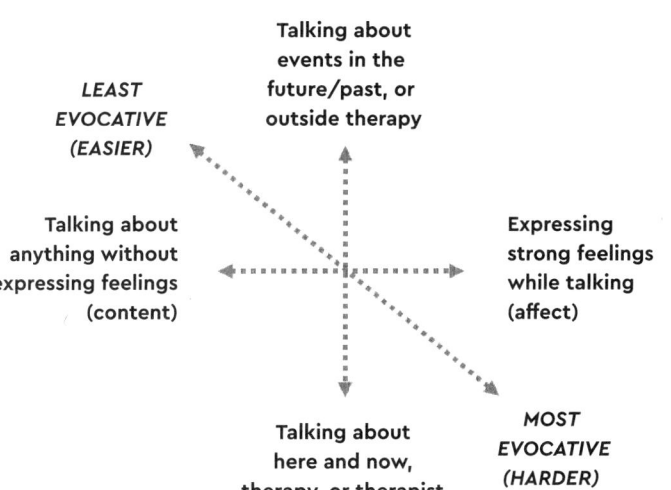

Note. Figure created by Jason Whipple, PhD.

- The person playing the client can use the advanced client statements again with a more distressed voice (very angry, sad, sarcastic, etc.) or unpleasant facial expression. This should increase the emotional tone.

- The client can improvise new client statements with topics that are more evocative or make the therapist uncomfortable, such as expressing strong feelings or talking about the here-and-now, therapy, or the therapist (see Figure A.2).

> *Note.* The purpose of a deliberate practice session is not to get through all the client statements and therapist responses but rather to spend as much time as possible practicing at the correct difficulty level. This may mean that trainees repeat the same statements and responses many times, which is okay, as long as the difficulty remains at the "good challenge" level.

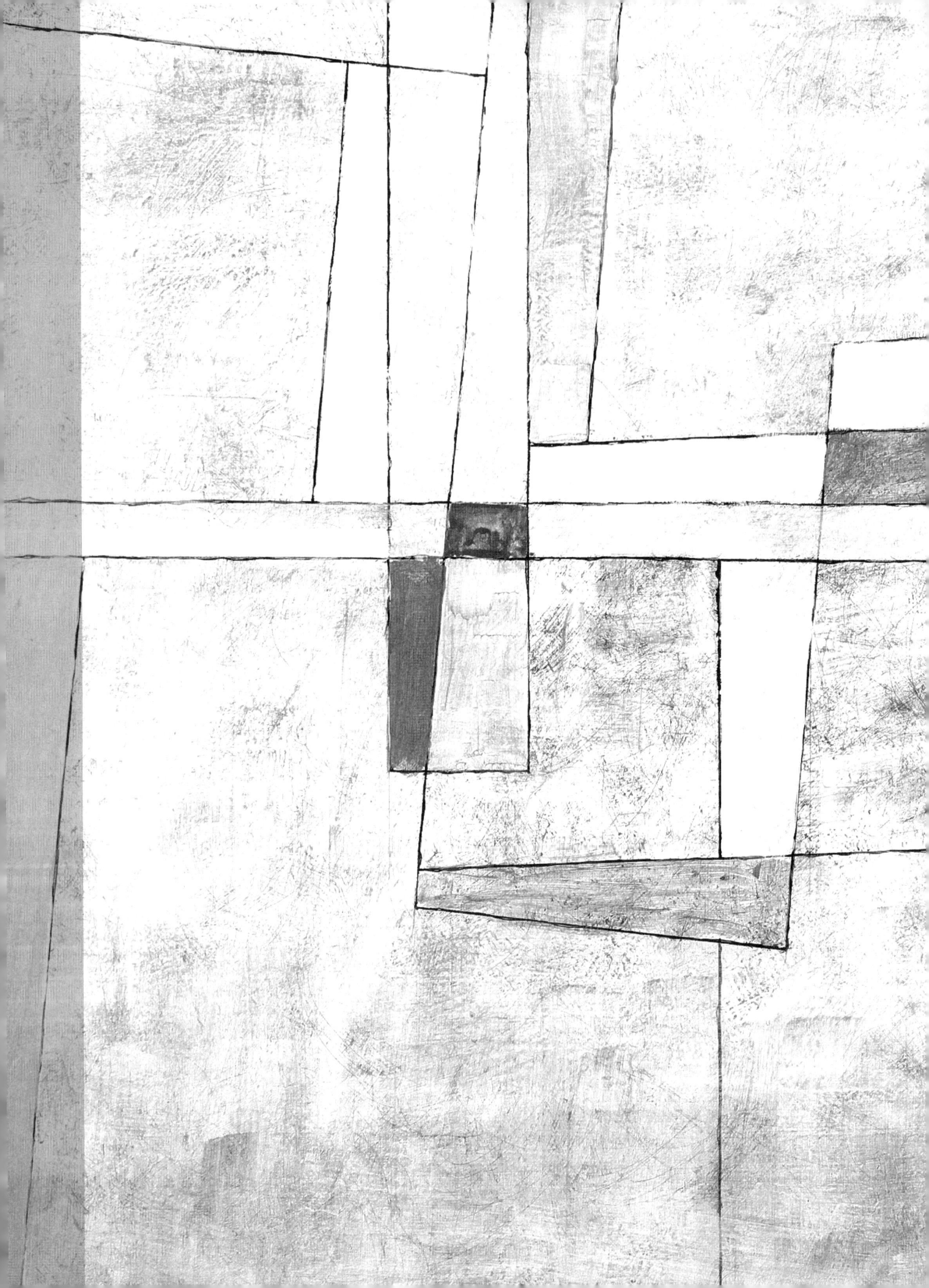

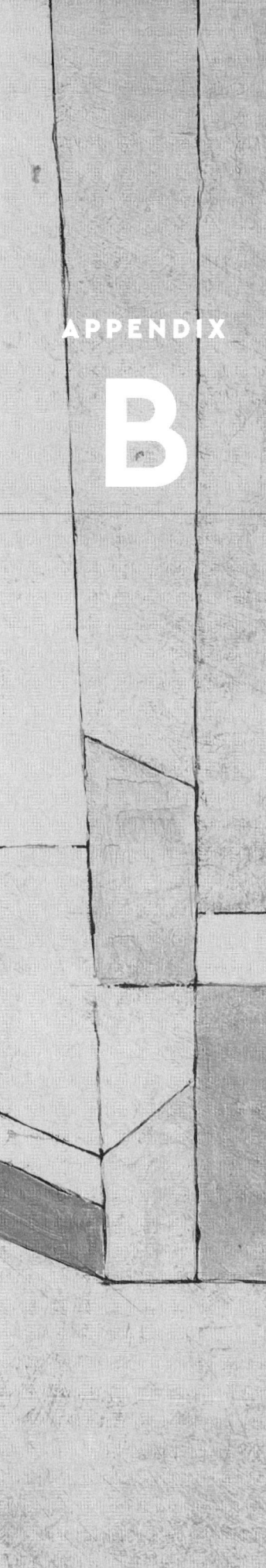

Deliberate Practice Diary Form

This book focuses on deliberate practice methods that involve active, live engagement between trainees and a supervisor. Importantly, deliberate practice can extend beyond these focused training sessions. For example, a trainee might read the client stimuli quietly or aloud and practice their responses independently between sessions with a supervisor. In such cases, it is important for the trainee to speak aloud rather than rehearse silently in one's head. Alternatively, two trainees can practice without the supervisor. Although the absence of a supervisor limits one source of feedback, the peer trainee who is playing the client can serve this role, as they can when a supervisor is present. Importantly, these additional deliberate practice opportunities are intended to take place between focused training sessions with a supervisor. To optimize the quality of the deliberate practice when conducted independently or without a supervisor, we have developed a Deliberate Practice Diary Form that can also be downloaded from the "Resources" tab online (https://www.apa.org/pubs/books/deliberate-practice-accelerated-experiential-dynamic-psychotherapy). This form provides a template for the trainee to record their experience of the deliberate practice activity and, ideally, will aid in the consolidation of learning. This form can also be used as part of the evaluation process with the supervisor but is not necessarily intended for that purpose, and trainees are certainly welcome to bring their experience with the independent practice into the next meeting with the supervisor.

Deliberate Practice Diary Form

Use this form to consolidate learnings from the deliberate practice exercises. Please protect your personal boundaries by only sharing information that you are comfortable disclosing.

Name: _____ Date: _____

Exercise: _____

Question 1. What was helpful or worked well this deliberate practice session? In what way?

Question 2. What was unhelpful or didn't go well this deliberate practice session? In what way?

Question 3. What did you learn about yourself, your current skills, and skills you'd like to keep improving? Feel free to share any details, but only those you are comfortable disclosing.

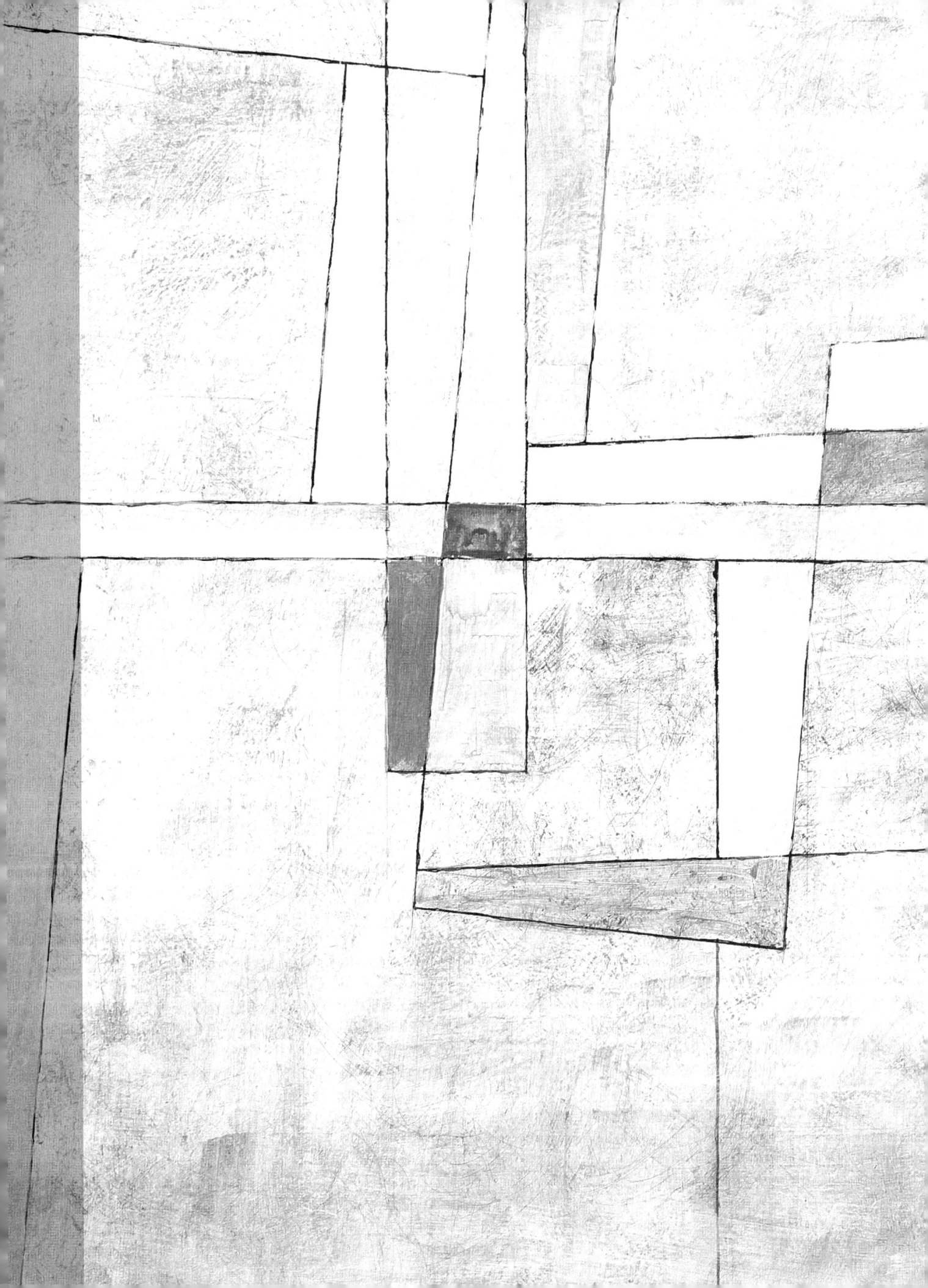

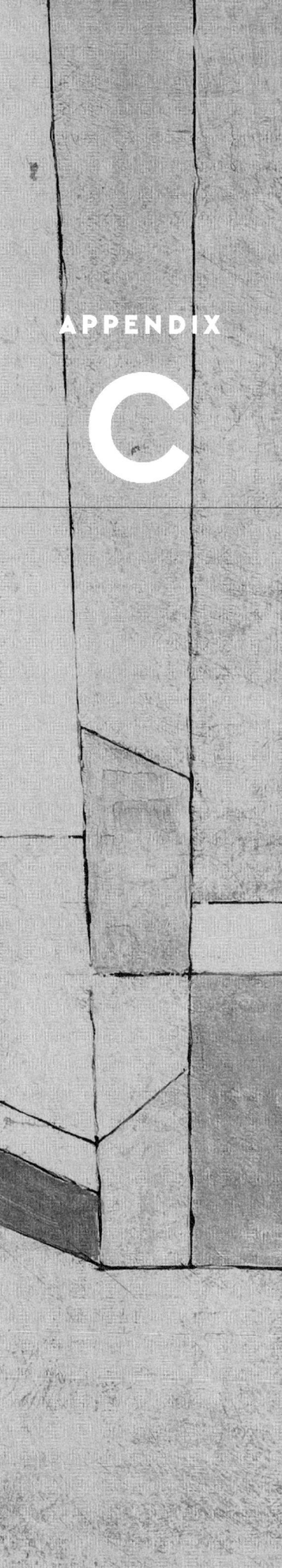

Sample Accelerated Experiential Dynamic Psychotherapy Syllabus With Embedded Deliberate Practice Exercises

Course Description

This course teaches theory, principles, and essential skills of accelerated experiential dynamic psychotherapy (AEDP). As a course with both didactic and practicum elements, it will review the theory and implementation of AEDP psychotherapy change processes, and foster the use of deliberate practice to enable students to acquire 12 key AEDP skills.

Course Objectives

Students who complete this course will be able to

1. Describe the theory, clinical practice, and skills of AEDP
2. Apply the principles of deliberate practice for career-long clinical skill development
3. Demonstrate key AEDP skills
4. Evaluate how they can fit AEDP skills into their developing therapeutic framework
5. Use AEDP with clients from diverse cultural backgrounds
6. Describe the ways in which AEDP uses interventions that are part of an evidence-based practice

Format of Class

Classes are 3 hours long. Course time is split evenly between learning and experiencing AEDP theory and acquiring AEDP skills. AEDP is an experiential, relational model and as such the course and class format will focus on experiential, relational, interactive learning:

Videos, Experiential Exercises, and Class Discussion: Each week, there will be 1.5 hours of interactive learning focusing on experiencing AEDP theory and acquiring knowledge of the related research. We prefer interactive, experiential learning over lecture.

AEDP Skills Lab: Each week there will be one AEDP skills lab for 1.5 hours. Skills Labs are for practicing AEDP skills using the exercises in this book. The exercises use therapy simulations (role plays) with the following goals:

1. Build trainees' skill and confidence for using AEDP skills with real clients.
2. Provide a space for experimenting with different therapeutic interventions, without fear of making mistakes.

Date	Lecture and Discussion	Skills Lab	Homework (to do before class)
Week 1	Introduction to AEDP theory and clinical practice Triangle of experience Four-state model	**Watch & Discuss:** APA video Fosha & Levenson (2016)	Fosha (2021) Kranz (2021) Prenn (2011) Check out exercises on the Sentio University site: https://sentio.org/
Week 2	Moment-to-moment tracking **Watch & Discuss** Dog video: https://www.youtube.com/watch?v=B8ISzf2pryI Discuss Fosha interview	Exercise 1: Moment-to-Moment Tracking **Watch & Discuss:** Watch a video of therapy session with sound off	Hanakawa (2021) Fosha interview [Video] (Fosha & Welling, 2011)
Week 3	Exploring and staying with physical experience Review triangle of experience States 1 and 2	Exercise 2: Exploring and Staying With Physical Experience	Hendel (n.d.) Read and watch two of the video links provided Hendel (2016, Chapter 1)
Week 4	We are in this together: undoing aloneness	Exercise 3: Undoing Aloneness	Lipton & Fosha (2011) Fosha (2005) Pando-Mars (2016)
Week 5	Affirming	Exercise 4: Affirming	Medley (2021b)
Week 6	Self-involving self-disclosure Use of the self in AEDP	Exercise 5: Self-Involving Self-Disclosure	Prenn (2009)
Week 7	Self-revealing self-disclosure Use of the self in AEDP	Exercise 6: Self-Revealing Self-Disclosure	Iwakabe & Conceição (2014)
Week 8	Metaprocessing	Exercise 7: Metaprocessing	Fosha & Thoma (2020)
Week 9	Working with anxiety Review triangle of experience	Exercise 8: Working With Anxiety	Russell (2021)
Week 10	Affirmative work with defenses	Exercise 9: Affirmative Work With Defenses	Hendel (2016; Chapters 5 and 6)
Week 11	Initiating portrayals	Exercise 10: Initiating Portrayals	Medley (2021a) Prenn (2010) Lamagna & Gleiser (2007)
Week 12	Privileging transformance strivings	Exercise 11: Privileging Transformance Strivings	Fosha (2017b)
Week 13	Metatherapeutic processing	Exercise 12: Metatherapeutic Processing	Fosha et al. (2019) Yeung (2021) Iwakabe & Conceição (2016)
Week 14	Putting it together	Exercise 13: Annotated AEDP Practice Session Transcript	Prenn & Halliday (2020) Harrison (2020) Blimling (2019a)
Week 15	Putting it all together	Exercise 14: Mock AEDP Sessions	Lipton (2020) Russell & Fosha (2008)

3. Provide plenty of opportunity to explore and "try on" different AEDP interventions, so trainees can ultimately discover their own personal, unique AEDP voice and style.

Mock Sessions: Once in the semester (Week 15), trainees will do a psychotherapy mock session in the AEDP skills lab. In contrast to highly structured and repetitive deliberate practice exercises, a psychotherapy mock session is an unstructured and improvised role-play therapy session. Mock sessions allow trainees

1. to practice using AEDP skills responsively,
2. to experiment with clinical decision making in an unscripted context,
3. to discover their personal therapeutic style, and
4. to build endurance for working with real clients.

Homework

Homework will be assigned each week and include reading and watching videos. As an option, trainees could also add 1 hour of skills practice with an assigned practice partner, particularly if they found a skill challenging. Trainees will complete the Deliberate Practice Reaction Form, as well as the Deliberate Practice Diary Form, for themselves as a self-evaluation tool.

Writing Assignments

Students are to write a paper due the last day of class. The instructor will choose the topic. The following are three possibilities:

1. Using one of the mock therapy profiles from Exercise 14, construct a partial transcript of an imagined session. The transcript must include at least nine of the 12 skills from this book, identified within the transcripted material (5–10 pages).

2. Using one of the mock therapy profiles from Exercise 14, video yourself with a partner. Go back over the video pretending you are your supervisor and list the observations you would make about your use of deliberate practice skills (5–10 pages).

3. Write a deliberate practice exercise on an AEDP skill not described in this book. Your write-up should include a short introduction to the skill, skill criteria, and three examples, using the format outlined in this book (3–4 pages). AEDP readings are a rich source of ideas for possible additional skills. If you are unsure, feel free to check with the instructor.

Multicultural and Social Orientation

This course is taught in a multicultural context, defined as "how the cultural worldviews, values, and beliefs of the client and therapist interact and influence one another to co-create a relational experience that is in the spirit of healing" (Davis et al., 2018, p. 90). Core features of the multicultural orientation include cultural comfort, humility, and responding to cultural opportunities (or previously missed opportunities). The stance and strategies of AEDP are well suited to notice, explore and make explicit the influence of cultural and social variables within the therapeutic dyadic. So many skills that AEDP uses (particularly self-disclosure, moment-to-moment tracking, and meta-processing which all work to make the implicit explicit) work to traverse perceived social and power dynamics (Fosha, 2018). Thus, AEDP incorporates a multicultural orientation (e.g., Gonzalez, 2018a, 2018b; Iwakabe, 2018; Skean, 2018) within its theory and practice. Medley (2021a, 2021b) has added the "triangle of social experience" to the AEDP metapsychology to facilitate an understanding of how institutional and interrelational stereotypes based on race, sexual orientation, gender, religion, class, age, size, and ability impact client–therapist dynamics and the process of healing.

Throughout this course, students are encouraged to reflect on their own cultural and social identities and improve their ability to attune with their clients' interlocking identities (Hook et al., 2017). For further guidance on this topic and deliberate practice exercises to improve multicultural skills, see the book *Deliberate Practice in Multicultural Therapy* (Harris et al., 2024).

Vulnerability, Privacy, and Boundaries

This course is aimed at developing AEDP skills, self-awareness, and interpersonal skills in an experiential framework and as relevant to clinical work. This course is not psychotherapy or a substitute for psychotherapy. Students should interact at a level of self-disclosure that is personally comfortable and helpful to their own learning. Although becoming aware of internal emotional and psychological processes is necessary for a therapist's development, it is not necessary to reveal all that information to the trainer. It is important for students to sense their own level of safety and privacy. Students are not evaluated on the level of material that they choose to reveal in the class.

In accordance with the *Ethical Principles of Psychologists and Code of Conduct* (American Psychological Association, 2017), **students are not required to disclose personal information.** Because this class is about developing both interpersonal and AEDP competence, following are some important points so that students are fully informed as they make choices to self-disclose:

- Students choose how much, when, and what to disclose. Students are not penalized for the choice not to share personal information.

- The learning environment is susceptible to group dynamics much like any other group space, and therefore students may be asked to share their observations and experiences of the class environment with the singular goal of fostering a more inclusive and productive learning environment. AEDP's metaprocessing (Exercise 7) and metatherapeutic processing (Exercise 12) skills are particularly useful in this context.

Confidentiality

To promote a safe learning environment that is respectful of client and therapist information and diversity and to foster open and vulnerable conversation in class, students are required to agree to strict confidentiality within and outside of the instruction setting.

Description Versus Evaluation

Self-Evaluation: At the end of the semester (Week 15), trainees will perform a self-evaluation. This will help trainees track their progress and identify areas for further development. The Guidance for Trainees section in Chapter 3 of this book highlights potential areas of focus for self-evaluation. Self-evaluation is very much in keeping with the AEDP philosophy of self-discovery.

Description Versus Evaluation: The stance of the AEDP is in favor of description rather than evaluation. "The word *evaluation* holds an anticipation of criticism and judgment. When we substitute the word *description* in its place, we are more aligned with our way of working" (Prenn & Fosha, 2017, p. 114). We invite the teacher of this course to consider giving continuous formative feedback rather than only a single, separate, summative course-end evaluation. This isn't to say that the teacher only gives positive feedback. "Limiting our feedback to praise only ultimately does not create safety" in the classroom (Prenn & Fosha, 2017, p. 116).

Grading Criteria

As designed, students would be accountable for the level and quality of their performance in the following:

- Class discussion and participation (25% of grade)
- The Skills Lab exercises (25% of grade)
- Self-evaluation based on coaching feedback (25% of grade)
- Final paper (25% of grade)

Required Readings and Resources

Blimling, G. P. (2019). The effect of integrating music listening with an attachment and affective-focused short-term psychotherapy in an individual with relational trauma: The case of "James." *Pragmatic Case Studies in Psychotherapy, 15*(2), 116–166. https://doi.org/10.14713/pcsp.v15i2.2051

Fosha, D. (2005). Emotion, true self, true other, core state: Toward a clinical theory of affective change process. *Psychoanalytic Review, 92*(4), 513–552. https://doi.org/10.1521/prev.2005.92.4.513

Fosha, D. (2017). How to be a transformational therapist: AEDP harnesses innate healing affects to rewire experience and accelerate transformation. In J. Loizzo, M. Neale, & E. Wolf (Eds.), *Advances in contemplative psychotherapy: Accelerating transformation* (pp. 204–219). W.W. Norton & Company. https://doi.org/10.4324/9781315630045-18

Fosha, D. (2021). Introduction: AEDP after 20 years. In D. Fosha (Ed.), *Undoing aloneness & the transformation of suffering into flourishing: AEDP 2.0* (pp. 3–23). American Psychological Association. https://doi.org/10.1037/0000232-001

Fosha, D. (Guest Expert), & Levenson, H. (Host). (2016). *Accelerated experiential dynamic psychotherapy (AEDP) supervision* [Video]. American Psychological Association. https://www.apa.org/pubs/videos/4310958

Fosha, D., & Thoma, N. (2020). Metatherapeutic processing supports the emergence of flourishing in psychotherapy. *Psychotherapy, 57*(3), 323–339. https://doi.org/10.1037/pst0000289

Fosha, D., Thoma, N., & Yeung, D. (2019). Transforming emotional suffering into flourishing: Metatherapeutic processing of positive affect as a trans-theoretical vehicle for change. *Counselling Psychology Quarterly, 32*(3–4), 563–593. https://doi.org/10.1080/09515070.2019.1642852

Fosha, D., & Welling, H. (Host). (2011). *Interview with Diana Fosha* [Video]. https://www.youtube.com/watch?v=bUnlArnZ96w

Hanakawa, Y. (2021). What just happened? and What is happening now? The art and science of moment-to-moment tracking in AEDP. In D. Fosha (Ed.), *Undoing aloneness & the transformation of suffering into flourishing: AEDP 2.0* (pp. 107–131). American Psychological Association. https://doi.org/10.1037/0000232-005

Harrison, R. L. (2020). Termination in 16-session accelerated experiential dynamic psycho-therapy (AEDP): Together in how we say goodbye. *Psychotherapy: Theory, Research, & Practice*, *57*(4), 531–547. https://doi.org/10.1037/pst0000343

Hendel, H. (n.d.). *What is the change triangle?* https://www.hilaryjacobshendel.com/what-is-the-change-triangle-c18dd

Hendel, H. (2016). *It's not always depression. Working with the change triangle to listen to the body, discover core emotions and connect to your authentic self.* Random House.

Iwakabe, S., & Conceição, N. (2014, June). *Therapist self-disclosure and therapist transfor-mation: A qualitative study on AEDP therapists' working with immediate experience.* Presentation given at the annual meeting of the Society for Psychotherapy Research, Copenhagen, Denmark.

Iwakabe, S., & Conceição, N. (2016). Metatherapeutic processing as a change-based therapeutic immediacy task: Building an initial process model using a task-analytic research strategy. *Journal of Psychotherapy Integration*, *26*(3), 230–247. https://doi.org/10.1037/int0000016

Kranz, K. (2021). The first session in AEDP: Harnessing transformance and cocreating a secure attachment. In D. Fosha (Ed.), *Undoing aloneness & the transformation of suffering into flourishing: AEDP 2.0* (pp. 53–79). American Psychological Association. https://doi.org/10.1037/0000232–003

Lamagna, J., & Gleiser, K. (2007). Building a secure internal attachment: An intra-relational approach to ego strengthening and emotional processing with chronically traumatized clients. *Journal of Trauma and Dissociation*, *8*(1), 25–52. https://doi.org/10.1300/J229v08n01_03

Lipton, B. (2020). The being is the doing: The foundational place of therapeutic presence in AEDP. *Transformance: The AEDP Journal*, *10*(4). https://aedpinstitute.org/the-therapeutic-presence-issue-liptonthe-being-is-the-doing/

Lipton, B., & Fosha, D. (2011). Attachment as a transformative process in AEDP: Operationalizing the intersection of attachment theory and affective neuroscience. *Journal of Psychotherapy Integration*, *21*(3), 253–279. https://doi.org/10.1037/a0025421

Medley, B. (2021a). Portrayals in work with emotion in AEDP. In D. Fosha (Ed.), *Undoing alone-ness & the transformation of suffering into flourishing: AEDP 2.0* (pp. 217–240). American Psychological Association. https://doi.org/10.1037/0000232-009

Medley, B. (2021b). Recovering the true self: Affirmative therapy, attachment, and AEDP in psychotherapy with gay men. *Journal of Psychotherapy Integration*, *31*(4), 383–402. https://doi.org/10.1037/int0000132

Pando-Mars, K. (2016). Tailoring AEDP Interventions to attachment style. *Transformance: The AEDP Journal*, *6*(2), 1–91.

Prenn, N. (2009). I second that emotion! On self-disclosure and its metaprocessing. In A. Bloomgarden & R. B. Mennuti (Eds.), *Psychotherapist revealed: Therapists speak about self-disclosure in psychotherapy* (pp. 85–99). Routledge/Taylor Francis Group.

Prenn, N. (2010). Transformance: Setting transformance into action: The AEDP protocol. *Trans-formance: The AEDP Journal*, *1*(1). https://aedpinstitute.org/transformance/how-to-set-transformance-into-action/

Prenn, N. (2011). Mind the gap: AEDP interventions translating attachment theory into clinical practice. *Journal of Psychotherapy Integration*, *21*(3), 308–329. https://doi.org/10.1037/a0025491

Prenn, N., & Halliday, K. (2020). See me, feel me: An AEDP toolbox for creating therapeutic presence online. *Transformance: The AEDP Journal*, *10*(6). https://aedpinstitute.org/transformance-volume-10-therapeutic-presence-halliday-prenn/

Russell, E. (2021). Agency, will, and desire as core affective experience. In D. Fosha (Ed.), *Undoing aloneness & the transformation of suffering into flourishing: AEDP 2.0* (pp. 241–265). American Psychological Association. https://doi.org/10.1037/0000232-010

Russell, E., & Fosha, D. (2008). Transformational affects and core state in AEDP: The emergence and consolidation of joy, hope, gratitude, and confidence in (the solid goodness of) the self. *Journal of Psychotherapy Integration*, *18*(2), 167–190. https://doi.org/10.1037/1053-0479.18.2.167

Yeung, D. (2021). What went right? What happens in the brain during AEDP's metatherapeutic processing. In D. Fosha (Ed.), *Undoing aloneness & the transformation of suffering into flourishing: AEDP 2.0* (pp. 349–376). American Psychological Association. https://doi.org/10.1037/0000232-014

Supplemental Readings

Fosha, D. (2000a). Meta-therapeutic processes and the affects of transformation: Affirmation and the healing affects. *Journal of Psychotherapy Integration, 10,* 71–97. https://doi.org/10.1023/A:1009422511959

Fosha, D. (2000b). *The transforming power of affect. A model for accelerated change.* Basic Books.

Fosha, D. (2001). The dyadic regulation of affect. *Journal of Clinical Psychology/In Session, 57*(2), 227–242. https://doi.org/10.1002/1097-4679(200102)57:2%3C227::AID-JCLP8%3E3.0.CO;2-1

Fosha, D. (2002). The activation of affective change processes in AEDP (accelerated experiential-dynamic psychotherapy). In J. J. Magnavita (Ed.), *Comprehensive handbook of psychotherapy: Vol. 1. Psychodynamic and object relations psychotherapies* (pp. 309–344). John Wiley & Sons.

Fosha, D. (2003). Dyadic regulation and experiential work with emotion and relatedness in trauma and disordered attachment. In M. F. Solomon & D. J. Siegel (Eds.), *Healing trauma: Attachment, mind, body, and brain* (pp. 221–281). W.W. Norton & Company.

Fosha, D. (2004a). Brief integrative psychotherapy comes of age: A commentary. *Journal of Psychotherapy Integration, 14*(1), 66–92. https://doi.org/10.1037/1053-0479.14.1.66

Fosha, D. (2004b). "Nothing that feels bad is ever the last step:" The role of positive emotions in experiential work with difficult emotional experiences. *Clinical Psychology and Psychotherapy, 11*(1), 30–43. https://doi.org/10.1002/cpp.390

Fosha, D. (2009). Emotion and recognition at work: Energy, vitality, pleasure, truth, desire, and the emergent phenomenology of transformational experience. In D. Fosha, D. J. Siegel, & M. F. Solomon (Eds.), *The healing power of emotion: Affective neuroscience, development, & clinical practice* (pp. 173–203). W.W. Norton & Company.

Fosha, D. (2017). Something more than "something more than interpretation": AEDP works the experiential edge of transformational experience to transform the internal working model. In S. Lord (Ed.), *Moments of meeting in psychoanalysis: Interaction and change in the therapeutic encounter* (pp. 267–292). Routledge/Taylor Francis Group.

Fosha, D., Coleman, J., Iwakabe, S., Gretton, H., & Owen, J. (2024). The development of the Moments of Flourishing Experience Scale (MFES): A multidimensional scale to measure positive affect based flourishing state experiences. *Counselling Psychology Quarterly.* Advance online publication. https://doi.org/10.1080/09515070.2024.2377167

Frederick, R. (2009). *Living like you mean it: Use the wisdom and power of your emotions to get the life you really want.* Jossey-Bass.

Frederick, R. (2021). Neuroplasticity in action: Rewiring internal working models of attachment. In D. Fosha (Ed.), *Undoing aloneness and the transformation of suffering into flourishing: AEDP 2.0* (pp. 189–216). American Psychological Association. https://doi.org/10.1037/0000232-008

Medley, B. (2024). Accelerated experiential dynamic psychotherapy: A model of change and transformation. In E. Seinreich & L. Straussner (Eds.) *Experiential therapies for the treatment of trauma.* Routledge/Taylor Francis Group. https://doi.org/10.1037/int0000132

Pando-Mars, K. (2021). Using AEDP's representational schemas to orient the therapist's attunement and engagement. In D. Fosha (Ed.), *Undoing aloneness and the transformation of suffering into flourishing: AEDP 2.0* (pp. 159–186). American Psychological Association. https://doi.org/10.1037/0000232-007

Tunnell, G. (2006). An affirmational approach to treating gay male couples. *Group, 30*(2), 133–151.

Tunnell, G. (2023). "Unequivocal Affirmation" of True Self in 16-session AEDP with gay men: Using relational metaprocessing to increase receptive affective capacity. *Transformance: The AEDP Journal.* https://aedpinstitute.org/transformance/unequivocal-affirmation-of-true-self-in-16-session-aedp-with-gay-menusing-relational-metaprocessing-to-increase-receptive-affective-capacity-gil-tunnel-phd-volume-11-issue-1/

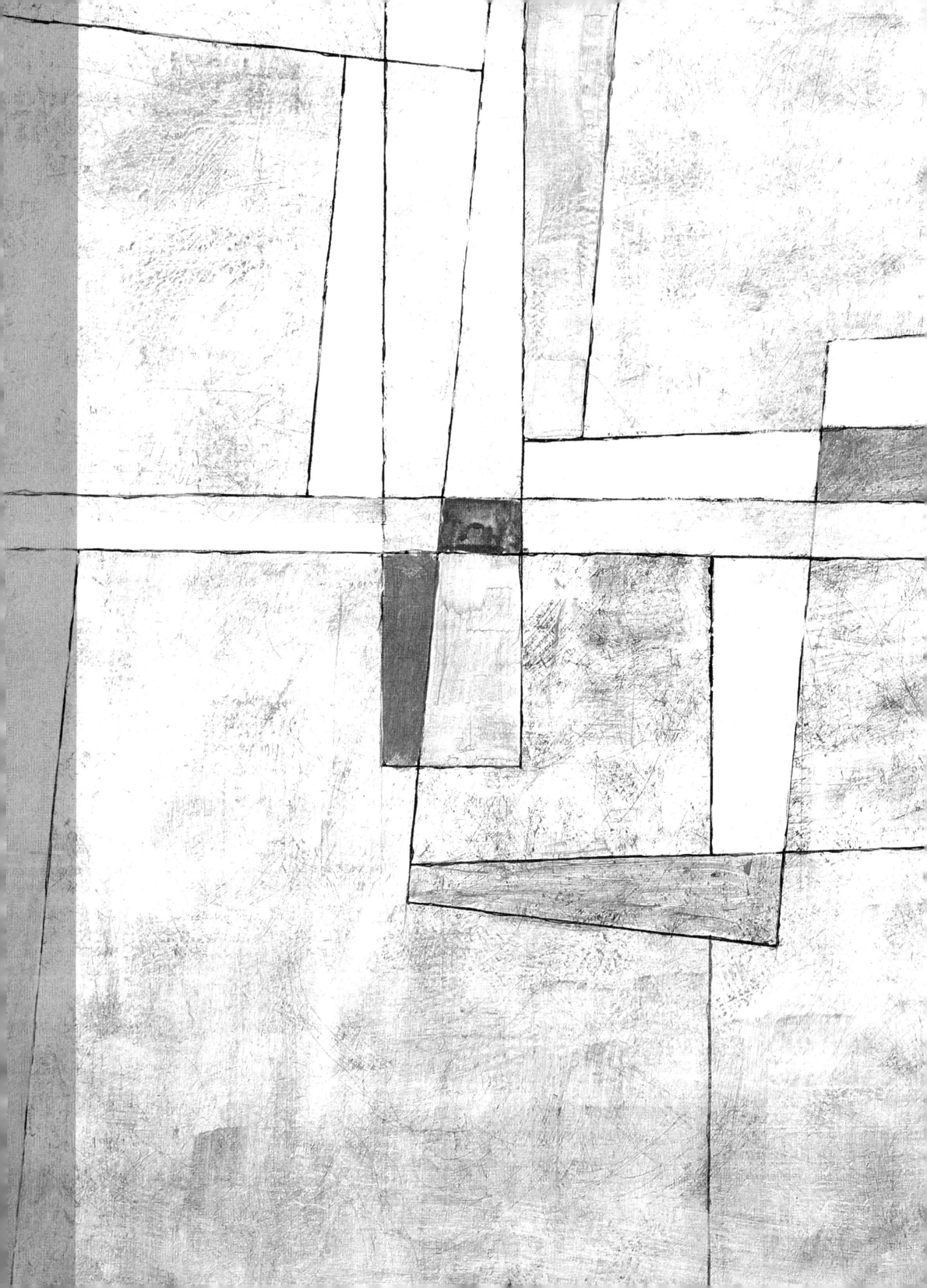

References

American Psychological Association. (2017). *Ethical principles of psychologists and code of conduct* (2002, Amended June 1, 2010, and January 1, 2017). https://www.apa.org/ethics/code/

Anderson, T., Ogles, B. M., Patterson, C. L., Lambert, M. J., & Vermeersch, D. A. (2009). Therapist effects: Facilitative interpersonal skills as a predictor of therapist success. *Journal of Clinical Psychology*, *65*(7), 755–768. https://doi.org/10.1002/jclp.20583

Bailey, R. J., & Ogles, B. M. (2019, August 1). Common factors as a therapeutic approach: What is required? *Practice Innovations*, *4*(4), 241–254. https://doi.org/10.1037/pri0000100

Barlow, D. H. (2010). Negative effects from psychological treatments: A perspective. *American Psychologist*, *65*(1), 13–20. https://doi.org/10.1037/a0015643

Bennett-Levy, J. (2019). Why therapists should walk the talk: The theoretical and empirical case for personal practice in therapist training and professional development. *Journal of Behavior Therapy and Experimental Psychiatry*, *62*, 133–145. https://doi.org/10.1016/j.jbtep.2018.08.004

Bennett-Levy, J., & Finlay-Jones, A. (2018). The role of personal practice in therapist skill development: A model to guide therapists, educators, supervisors and researchers. *Cognitive Behaviour Therapy*, *47*(3), 185–205. https://doi.org/10.1080/16506073.2018.1434678

Blimling, G. P. (2019a). The effect of integrating music listening with an attachment and affective-focused short-term psychotherapy in an individual with relational trauma: The case of "James." *Pragmatic Case Studies in Psychotherapy*, *15*(2), 116–166.

Blimling, G. P. (2019b). Facing the music: Further thoughts on integrating music into psychotherapy. *Pragmatic Case Studies in Psychotherapy*, *15*(2), 206–213. https://doi.org/10.14713/pcsp.v15i2.2055

Bohart, A. C., & Wade, A. G. (2013). The client in psychotherapy. In M. J. Lambert (Ed.), *Bergin and Garfield's handbook of psychotherapy and behavior change* (5th ed., pp. 13–43). John Wiley & Sons.

Bollas, C. (1987). *The shadow of the object: Psychoanalysis of the unthought known*. Columbia University Press.

Bugatti, M., & Boswell, J. F. (2016). Clinical errors as a lack of context responsiveness. *Psychotherapy: Theory, Research, & Practice*, *53*(3), 262–267. https://doi.org/10.1037/pst0000080

Castonguay, L. G., Goldfried, M. R., Wiser, S., Raue, P. J., & Hayes, A. M. (1996). Predicting the effect of cognitive therapy for depression: A study of unique and common factors. *Journal of Consulting and Clinical Psychology*, *64*(3), 497–504. https://doi.org/10.1037/0022-006X.64.3.497

Coker, J. (1990). *How to practice jazz*. Jamey Aebersold.

Cook, R. (2005). *It's about that time: Miles Davis on and off record*. Atlantic Books.

Csikszentmihalyi, M. (1997). *Finding flow: The psychology of engagement with everyday life.* HarperCollins.

Davis, D. E., DeBlaere, C., Owen, J., Hook, J. N., Rivera, D. P., Choe, E., Van Tongeren, D. R., Worthington, E. L., & Placeres, V. (2018). The multicultural orientation framework: A narrative review. *Psychotherapy: Theory, Research, & Practice, 55*(1), 89–100. https://doi.org/10.1037/pst0000160

Ellis, M. V., Berger, L., Hanus, A. E., Ayala, E. E., Swords, B. A., & Siembor, M. (2014). Inadequate and harmful clinical supervision: Testing a revised framework and assessing occurrence. *The Counseling Psychologist, 42*(4), 434–472. https://doi.org/10.1177/0011000013508656

Ericsson, K. A. (2003). Development of elite performance and deliberate practice: An update from the perspective of the expert performance approach. In J. L. Starkes & K. A. Ericsson (Eds.), *Expert performance in sports: Advances in research on sport expertise* (pp. 49–83). Human Kinetics.

Ericsson, K. A. (2004). Deliberate practice and the acquisition and maintenance in medicine and related domains: Invited address. *Academic Medicine, 79*(Suppl.), S70–S81. https://doi.org/10.1097/00001888-200410001-00022

Ericsson, K. A. (2006). The influence of experience and deliberate practice on the development of superior expert performance. In K. A. Ericsson, N. Charness, P. J. Feltovich, & R. R. Hoffman (Eds.), *The Cambridge handbook of expertise and expert performance* (pp. 683–704). Cambridge University Press. https://doi.org/10.1017/CBO9780511816796.038

Ericsson, K. A., Hoffman, R. R., Kozbelt, A., & Williams, A. M. (Eds.). (2018). *The Cambridge handbook of expertise and expert performance* (2nd ed.). Cambridge University Press. https://doi.org/10.1017/9781316480748

Ericsson, K. A., Krampe, R. T., & Tesch-Römer, C. (1993). The role of deliberate practice in the acquisition of expert performance. *Psychological Review, 100*(3), 363–406. https://doi.org/10.1037/0033-295X.100.3.363

Ericsson, K. A., & Pool, R. (2016). *Peak: Secrets from the new science of expertise.* Houghton Mifflin Harcourt.

Faerstein, I., Levenson, H., & Lee, A. C. (2016). Validation of a fidelity scale for accelerated-experiential dynamic psychotherapy. *Journal of Psychotherapy Integration, 26*(2), 172–185. https://doi.org/10.1037/int0000020

Fisher, R. P., & Craik, F. I. M. (1977). Interaction between encoding and retrieval operations in cued recall. *Journal of Experimental Psychology: Human Learning and Memory, 3*(6), 701–711. https://doi.org/10.1037/0278-7393.3.6.701

Fosha, D. (2000). *The transforming power of affect: A model for accelerated change.* Basic Books.

Fosha, D. (2001). The dyadic regulation of affect. *Journal of Clinical Psychology, 57*(2), 227–242. https://doi.org/10.1002/1097-4679(200102)57:2<227::AID-JCLP8>3.0.CO;2-1

Fosha, D. (2002). The activation of affective change processes in AEDP (accelerated experiential-dynamic psychotherapy). In J. J. Magnavita (Ed.), *Comprehensive handbook of psychotherapy: Vol. 1. Psychodynamic and object relations psychotherapies* (pp. 309–344). John Wiley & Sons.

Fosha, D. (2003). Dyadic regulation and experiential work with emotion and relatedness in trauma and disordered attachment. In M. F. Solomon & D. J. Siegel (Eds.), *Healing trauma: Attachment, mind, body, and brain* (pp. 221–281). W.W. Norton & Company.

Fosha, D. (2004a). Brief integrative psychotherapy comes of age: Reflections. *Journal of Psychotherapy Integration, 14*(1), 66–92. https://doi.org/10.1037/1053-0479.14.1.66

Fosha, D. (2004b). "Nothing that feels bad is ever the last step": The role of positive emotions in experiential work with difficult emotional experiences. *Clinical Psychology & Psychotherapy, 11*(1), 30–43. https://doi.org/10.1002/cpp.390

Fosha, D. (2005). Emotion, true self, true other, core state: Toward a clinical theory of affective change process. *Psychoanalytic Review, 92*(4), 513–551. https://doi.org/10.1521/prev.2005.92.4.513

Fosha, D. (2006). Quantum transformation in trauma and treatment: Traversing the crisis of healing change. *Journal of Clinical Psychology: In Session, 62*(5), 569–583.

Fosha, D. (2009). Emotion and recognition at work: Energy, vitality, pleasure, truth, desire, and the emergent phenomenology of transformational experience. In D. Fosha, D. J. Siegel, & M. F. Solomon (Eds.), *The healing power of emotion: Affective neuroscience, development, & clinical practice* (pp. 173–203). W.W. Norton & Company.

Fosha, D. (2013). Turbocharging the affects of healing and redressing the evolutionary tilt. In D. J. Siegel & Marion F. Solomon (Eds.), *Healing moments in psychotherapy* (pp. 129–168). W.W. Norton & Company.

Fosha, D. (2017a). How to be a transformational therapist: AEDP harnesses innate healing affects to rewire experience and accelerate transformation. In J. Loizzo, M. Neale, & E. Wolf (Eds.), *Advances in contemplative psychotherapy: Accelerating transformation* (pp. 204–219). W.W. Norton & Company. https://doi.org/10.4324/9781315630045-18

Fosha, D. (2017b). Something more than "something more than interpretation": AEDP works the experiential edge of transformational experience to transform the internal working model. In S. Lord (Ed.), *Moments of meeting in psychoanalysis: Interaction and change in the therapeutic encounter* (pp. 267–292). Routledge/Taylor Francis Group.

Fosha, D. (2018). Moment-to-moment guidance of clinical interventions by AEDP's healing-oriented, transformational phenomenology: Commentary on Vigoda Gonzalez's (2018) Case of "Rosa." *Pragmatic Case Studies in Psychotherapy*, 14(2), 87–114. https://doi.org/10.14713/pcsp.v14i2.2038

Fosha, D. (2021). Introduction: AEDP after 20 years. In D. Fosha (Ed.), *Undoing aloneness & the transformation of suffering into flourishing: AEDP 2.0* (pp. 3–23). American Psychological Association. https://doi.org/10.1037/0000232-001

Fosha, D., Coleman, J., Iwakabe, S., Gretton, H., & Owen, J. (2024). The development of the Moments of Flourishing Experience Scale (MFES): A multidimensional scale to measure positive affect based flourishing state experiences. *Counselling Psychology Quarterly*. Advance online publication. https://doi.org/10.1080/09515070.2024.2377167

Fosha, D. (Guest Expert), & Levenson, H. (Host). (2016). *Accelerated experiential dynamic psychotherapy (AEDP) supervision* [Video]. American Psychological Association. https://www.apa.org/pubs/videos/4310958

Fosha, D., & Thoma, N. (2020). Metatherapeutic processing supports the emergence of flourishing in psychotherapy. *Psychotherapy: Theory, Research, & Practice*, 57(3), 323–339. https://doi.org/10.1037/pst0000289

Fosha, D., Thoma, N., & Yeung, D. (2019). Transforming emotional suffering into flourishing: Metatherapeutic processing of positive affect as a trans-theoretical vehicle for change. *Counselling Psychology Quarterly*, 32(3–4), 563–593. https://doi.org/10.1080/09515070.2019.1642852

Fosha, D., & Welling, H. (Host). (2011). *Interview with Diana Fosha* [Video]. https://www.youtube.com/watch?v=bUnIArnZ96w

Frederick, R. (2009). *Living like you mean it: Use the wisdom and power of your emotions to get the life you really want*. Jossey-Bass.

Frederick, R. (2021). Neuroplasticity in action: Rewiring internal working models of attachment. In D. Fosha (Ed.), *Undoing aloneness and the transformation of suffering into flourishing: AEDP 2.0* (pp. 189–216). American Psychological Association. https://doi.org/10.1037/0000232-008

Fredrickson, B. L. (2001). The role of positive emotions in positive psychology: The broaden-and-build theory of positive emotions. *American Psychologist*, 56(3), 218–226. https://doi.org/10.1037/0003-066X.56.3.218

Geller, S. (2020). Cultivating therapeutic presence: Strengthening your clinical heart, mind and practice. *Transformance: The AEDP Journal*, 10. https://aedpinstitute.org/transformance/cultivating-therapeutic-presence-geller-volume-1preparing-prior-to-session/

Gladwell, M. (2008). *Outliers: The story of success*. Little, Brown & Company.

Glass, P., & Glass, I. (Interviewer). (2012, January 32). Ira Glass interviews his cousin, composer Philip Glass [Radio interview]. *Fresh Air*. NPR. Originally broadcast September 21, 1999. https://www.npr.org/2012/01/31/146092923/ira-glass-interviews-his-cousin-composer-philip-glass

Goldberg, S., Rousmaniere, T. G., Miller, S. D., Whipple, J., Nielsen, S. L., Hoyt, W., & Wampold, B. E. (2016). Do psychotherapists improve with time and experience? A longitudinal analysis of outcomes in a clinical setting. *Journal of Counseling Psychology*, *63*(1), 1–11. https://doi.org/10.1037/cou0000131

Goldman, R. N., Vaz, A., & Rousmaniere, T. (2021). *Deliberate practice in emotion-focused therapy*. American Psychological Association. https://doi.org/10.1037/0000227-000

Gonzalez, N. V. (2018a). The case of "Rosa": Reflections on the treatment of a survivor of relational trauma. *Pragmatic Case Studies in Psychotherapy*, *14*(1), 77–86. https://doi.org/10.14713/pcsp.v14i1.2035

Gonzalez, N. V. (2018b). The merits of integrating accelerated experiential dynamic psychotherapy and cultural competence strategies in the treatment of relational trauma: The case of "Rosa." *Pragmatic Case Studies in Psychotherapy*, *14*(1), 1–57. https://doi.org/10.14713/pcsp.v14i1.2032

Goodyear, R. K. (2015). Using accountability mechanisms more intentionally: A framework and its implications for training professional psychologists. *American Psychologist*, *70*(8), 736–743. https://doi.org/10.1037/a0039828

Goodyear, R. K., & Nelson, M. L. (1997). The major formats of psychotherapy supervision. In C. E. Watkins, Jr. (Ed.), *Handbook of psychotherapy supervision* (pp. 328–334). John Wiley & Sons.

Greenberg, L. S., & Goldman, R. L. (1988). Training in experiential therapy. *Journal of Consulting and Clinical Psychology*, *56*(5), 696–702. https://doi.org/10.1037/0022-006X.56.5.696

Greenberg, L. S., & Malcolm, W. (2002). Resolving unfinished business: Relating process to outcome. *Journal of Consulting and Clinical Psychology*, *70*(2), 406–416. https://doi.org/10.1037/0022-006X.70.2.406

Greenberg, L. S., Rice, L. N., & Elliot, R. (1993). *Facilitating emotional change: The moment-by-moment process*. Guilford Press.

Greenberg, L. S., & Watson, J. C. (2006). *Emotion-focused therapy for depression*. American Psychological Association.

Haggerty, G., & Hilsenroth, M. J. (2011). The use of video in psychotherapy supervision. *British Journal of Psychotherapy*, *27*(2), 193–210. https://doi.org/10.1111/j.1752-0118.2011.01232.x

Hanakawa, Y. (2021). What just happened? and What is happening now? The art and science of moment-to-moment tracking in AEDP. In D. Fosha (Ed.), *Undoing aloneness & the transformation of suffering into flourishing: AEDP 2.0* (pp. 107–131). American Psychological Association. https://doi.org/10.1037/0000232-005

Harris, J., Jin, J., Hoffman, S., Phan, S., Prout, T. A., Rousmaniere, T. G., & Vaz, A. (2024). *Deliberate practice in multicultural counseling*. American Psychological Association. https://doi.org/10.1037/0000357-000

Harrison, R. (2019). A bridge over troubled water: Commentary on Paul Blimling's case of "James" integrating music listening into AEDP. *Pragmatic Case Studies in Psychotherapy: PCSP*, *15*(2), 175–197. https://doi.org/10.14713/pcsp.v15i2.2053

Harrison, R. L. (2020). Termination in 16-session accelerated experiential dynamic psychotherapy (AEDP): Together in how we say goodbye. *Psychotherapy: Theory, Research, & Practice*, *57*(4), 531–547. https://doi.org/10.1037/pst0000343

Hatcher, R. L. (2015). Interpersonal competencies: Responsiveness, technique, and training in psychotherapy. *American Psychologist*, *70*(8), 747–757. https://doi.org/10.1037/a0039803

Hendel, H. (n.d.). *What is the change triangle?* https://www.hilaryjacobshendel.com/what-is-the-change-triangle-c18dd

Hendel, H. (2016). *It's not always depression: Working with the change triangle to listen to the body, discover core emotions, and connect to your authentic self*. Random House.

Henry, W. P., Strupp, H. H., Butler, S. F., Schacht, T. E., & Binder, J. L. (1993). Effects of training in time-limited dynamic psychotherapy: Changes in therapist behavior. *Journal of Consulting and Clinical Psychology*, *61*(3), 434–440. https://doi.org/10.1037/0022-006X.61.3.434

Hill, C. E., Kivlighan, D. M. I. I. I., Rousmaniere, T., Kivlighan, D. M., Jr., Gerstenblith, J. A., & Hillman, J. W. (2020). Deliberate practice for the skill of immediacy: A multiple case study of doctoral student therapists and clients. *Psychotherapy: Theory, Research, & Practice*, *57*(4), 587–597. https://doi.org/10.1037/pst0000247

Hill, C. E., & Knox, S. (2001). Self-disclosure. *Psychotherapy: Theory, Research, & Practice, 38*(4), 413–417. https://doi.org/10.1037/0033-3204.38.4.413

Hill, C. E., & Knox, S. (2013). Training and supervision in psychotherapy: Evidence for effective practice. In M. J. Lambert (Ed.), *Handbook of psychotherapy and behavior change* (6th ed., pp. 775–811). John Wiley & Sons.

Hook, J. N., Davis, D. D., Owen, J., & DeBlaere, C. (2017). *Cultural humility: Engaging diverse identities in therapy.* American Psychological Association Press. https://doi.org/10.1037/0000037-000

Iwakabe, S. (2018). Case studies in Accelerated Experiential Dynamic Psychotherapy (AEDP): Reflections on the case of "Rosa". *Pragmatic Case Studies in Psychotherapy, 14*(1), 58–68. https://doi.org/10.14713/pcsp.v14i1.2033

Iwakabe, S., & Conceição, N. (2014, June). *Therapist self-disclosure and therapist transformation: A qualitative study on AEDP therapists' working with immediate experience.* Presentation given at the annual meeting of the Society for Psychotherapy Research, Copenhagen, Denmark.

Iwakabe, S., & Conceição, N. (2016). Metatherapeutic processing as a change-based therapeutic immediacy task: Building an initial process model using a task-analytic research strategy. *Journal of Psychotherapy Integration, 26*(3), 230–247. https://doi.org/10.1037/int0000016

Iwakabe, S., Edlin, J., Fosha, D., Gretton, H., Joseph, A. J., Nunnink, S. E., Nakamura, K., & Thoma, N. C. (2020). The effectiveness of accelerated experiential dynamic psychotherapy (AEDP) in private practice settings: A transdiagnostic study conducted within the context of a practice-research network. *Psychotherapy: Theory, Research, & Practice, 57*(4), 548–561. https://doi.org/10.1037/pst0000344

Iwakabe, S., Edlin, J., Fosha, D., Thoma, N. C., Gretton, H., Joseph, A. J., & Nakamura, K. (2022). The long-term outcome of accelerated experiential dynamic psychotherapy: 6- and 12-month follow-up results. *Psychotherapy: Theory, Research, & Practice, 59*(3), 431–446. https://doi.org/10.1037/pst0000441

Jourard, S. M. (1971). *The transparent self.* Van Nostrand.

Kendall, P. C., & Beidas, R. S. (2007). Smoothing the trail for dissemination of evidence-based practices for youth: Flexibility within fidelity. *Professional Psychology, Research and Practice, 38*(1), 13–20. https://doi.org/10.1037/0735-7028.38.1.13

Kendall, P. C., & Frank, H. E. (2018). Implementing evidence-based treatment protocols: Flexibility within fidelity. *Clinical Psychology: Science and Practice, 25*(4), Article e12271. https://doi.org/10.1111/cpsp.12271

Knox, S., Hess, S. A., Petersen, D. A., & Hill, C. E. (1997). A qualitative analysis of client perceptions of the effects of helpful therapist self-disclosure in long-term therapy. *Journal of Counseling Psychology, 44*(3), 274–283. https://doi.org/10.1037/0022-0167.44.3.274

Koziol, L. F., & Budding, D. E. (2012). Procedural learning. In N. M. Seel (Ed.), *Encyclopedia of the sciences of learning* (pp. 2694–2696). Springer. https://doi.org/10.1007/978-1-4419-1428-6_670

Kranz, K. (2021). The first session in AEDP: Harnessing transformance and cocreating a secure attachment. In D. Fosha (Ed.), *Undoing aloneness & the transformation of suffering into flourishing: AEDP 2.0* (pp. 53–79). American Psychological Association. https://doi.org/10.1037/0000232-003

Lamagna, J., & Gleiser, K. A. (2007). Building a secure internal attachment: An intra-relational approach to ego strengthening and emotional processing with chronically traumatized clients. *Journal of Trauma & Dissociation, 8*(1), 25–52. https://doi.org/10.1300/J229v08n01_03

Lambert, M. J. (2010). Yes, it is time for clinicians to monitor treatment outcome. In B. L. Duncan, S. C. Miller, B. E. Wampold, & M. A. Hubble (Eds.), *Heart and soul of change: Delivering what works in therapy* (2nd ed., pp. 239–266). American Psychological Association. https://doi.org/10.1037/12075-008

Lee, A. C. (2015). *Building a model for metaprocessing: Exploration of a key change event in Accelerated Experiential Dynamic Psychotherapy (AEDP)* [Unpublished doctoral dissertation]. Wright Institute.

Levenson, H. (1995). *Time-limited dynamic psychotherapy: A guide to clinical practice.* American Psychological Association.

Levenson, H. (2017). *Brief dynamic therapy* (2nd ed.). American Psychological Association. https://doi.org/10.1037/0000043-000

Levenson, H., Fosha, D., & faculty members of the AEDP Institute. (2011). *The AEDP Knowledge and Competency Scale: Construction and psychometric properties* [Unpublished manuscript].

Levenson, H., Jinich, S., Vaz, A., & Rousmaniere, T. (2025). *Deliberate practice in emotionally focused couple therapy.* American Psychological Association. https://doi.org/10.1037/0000436-000

Lipton, B. (2020). The being is the doing: The foundational place of therapeutic presence in AEDP. *Transformance: The AEDP Journal, 10*(4). https://aedpinstitute.org/the-therapeutic-presence-issue-liptonthe-being-is-the-doing/

Lipton, B., & Fosha, D. (2011). Attachment as a transformative process in AEDP: Operationalizing the intersection of attachment theory and affective neuroscience. *Journal of Psychotherapy Integration, 21*(3), 253–279. https://doi.org/10.1037/a0025421

Markin, R. D., McCarthy, K. S., Fuhrmann, A., Yeung, D., & Gleiser, K. A. (2018). The process of change in accelerated experiential dynamic psychotherapy (AEDP): A case study analysis. *Journal of Psychotherapy Integration, 28*(2), 213–232. https://doi.org/10.1037/int0000084

Markman, K. D., & Tetlock, P. E. (2000). Accountability and close-call counterfactuals: The loser who nearly won and the winner who nearly lost. *Personality and Social Psychology Bulletin, 26*(10), 1213–1224. https://doi.org/10.1177/0146167200262004

Maroda, K. J. (1998). *Seduction, surrender, and transformation. Emotional engagement in the analytic process.* The Analytic Press.

McGaghie, W. C., Issenberg, S. B., Barsuk, J. H., & Wayne, D. B. (2014). A critical review of simulation-based mastery learning with translational outcomes. *Medical Education, 48*(4), 375–385. https://doi.org/10.1111/medu.12391

McLeod, J. (2017). Qualitative methods for routine outcome measurement. In T. G. Rousmaniere, R. Goodyear, D. D. Miller, & B. E. Wampold (Eds.), *The cycle of excellence: Using deliberate practice to improve supervision and training* (pp. 99–122). John Wiley & Sons. https://doi.org/10.1002/9781119165590.ch5

Medley, B. (2021a). Portrayals in work with emotion in AEDP. In D. Fosha (Ed.), *Undoing aloneness & the transformation of suffering into flourishing: AEDP 2.0* (pp. 217–240). American Psychological Association. https://doi.org/10.1037/0000232-009

Medley, B. (2021b). Recovering the true self: Affirmative therapy, attachment, and AEDP in psychotherapy with gay men. *Journal of Psychotherapy Integration, 31*(4), 383–402. https://doi.org/10.1037/int0000132

Miller, S. D., Hubble, M. A., & Chow, D. (2018). The question of expertise in psychotherapy. *Journal of Expertise, 1*(2), 121–129. https://journalofexpertise.org/articles/volume1_issue2/

Norcross, J. C., & Guy, J. D. (2005). The prevalence and parameters of personal therapy in the United States. In J. D. Geller, J. C. Norcross, & D. E. Orlinsky (Eds.), *The psychotherapist's own psychotherapy: Patient and clinician perspectives* (pp. 165–176). Oxford University Press.

Norcross, J. C., Lambert, M. J., & Wampold, B. E. (2019). *Psychotherapy relationships that work* (3rd ed.). Oxford University Press.

Notsu, H., Iwakabe, S., & Thoma, N. C. (2023). Enhancing working alliance through positive emotional experience: A cross-lag analysis. *Psychotherapy Research, 33*(3), 328–341. https://doi.org/10.1080/10503307.2022.2124893

Orlinsky, D. E., & Ronnestad, M. H. (2005). *How psychotherapists develop.* American Psychological Association.

Owen, J., & Hilsenroth, M. J. (2014). Treatment adherence: The importance of therapist flexibility in relation to therapy outcomes. *Journal of Counseling Psychology, 61*(2), 280–288. https://doi.org/10.1037/a0035753

Pally, R., & Olds, D. (2000). *How the brain actively constructs perceptions.* Routledge.

Pando-Mars, K. (2016). Tailoring AEDP Interventions to attachment style. *Transformance: The AEDP Journal, 6*(2), 1–91.

Pando-Mars, K. (2021). Using AEDP's representational schemas to orient the therapist's attunement and engagement. In D. Fosha (Ed.), *Undoing aloneness and the transformation of suffering into flourishing: AEDP 2.0* (pp. 159–186). American Psychological Association. https://doi.org/10.1037/0000232-007

Pando-Mars, K., & Fosha, D. (2025). *Healing relational trauma by tailoring treatment to patterns of attachment.* W.W. Norton & Company.

Prenn, N. (2009). I second that emotion! On self-disclosure and its metaprocessing. In A. Bloomgarden & R. B. Mennuti (Eds.), *Psychotherapist revealed: Therapists speak about self-disclosure in psychotherapy* (pp. 85–99). Routledge/Taylor Francis Group.

Prenn, N. (2010). Transformance: Setting transformance in action: The AEDP protocol. *Transformance: The AEDP Journal, 1*(1). https://aedpinstitute.org/transformance/how-to-set-transformance-into-action/

Prenn, N. (2011). Mind the gap: AEDP interventions translating attachment theory into clinical practice. *Journal of Psychotherapy Integration, 21*(3), 308–329. https://doi.org/10.1037/a0025491

Prenn, N., & Halliday, K. (2020). See me, feel me: An AEDP toolbox for creating therapeutic presence online. *Transformance: The AEDP Journal, 10*(6). https://aedpinstitute.org/transformance-volume-10-therapeutic-presence-halliday-prenn/

Prenn, N. C. N., & Fosha, D. (2017). *Supervision essentials for accelerated experiential dynamic psychotherapy.* American Psychological Association. https://doi.org/10.1037/0000016-000

Rousmaniere, T. G. (2016). *Deliberate practice for psychotherapists: A guide to improving clinical effectiveness.* Routledge/Taylor Francis Group. https://doi.org/10.4324/9781315472256

Rousmaniere, T. G. (2019). *Mastering the inner skills of psychotherapy: A deliberate practice handbook.* Gold Lantern Press.

Rousmaniere, T. G., Goodyear, R., Miller, S. D., & Wampold, B. E. (Eds.). (2017). *The cycle of excellence: Using deliberate practice to improve supervision and training.* John Wiley & Sons. https://doi.org/10.1002/9781119165590

Russell, E. (2007). *AEDP core training.* AEDP Training Institute.

Russell, E. (2021). Agency, will, and desire as core affective experience. In D. Fosha (Ed.), *Undoing aloneness & the transformation of suffering into flourishing: AEDP 2.0* (pp. 241–265). American Psychological Association. https://doi.org/10.1037/0000232-010

Russell, E., & Fosha, D. (2008). Transformational affects and core state in AEDP: The emergence and consolidation of joy, hope, gratitude, and confidence in (the solid goodness of) the self. *Journal of Psychotherapy Integration, 18*(2), 167–190. https://doi.org/10.1037/1053-0479.18.2.167

Schore, A. (2001). Effects of a secure attachment relationship on right brain development, affect regulation, and infant mental health. *Infant Mental Health Journal, 22*(1–2), 7–66. https://doi.org/10.1002/1097-0355(200101/04)22:1<7::AID-IMHJ2>3.0.CO;2-N

Schore, A. (2009). Right-brain regulation: An essential mechanism of development, trauma, dissociation, and psychotherapy. In D. Fosha, D. J. Siegel, & M. F. Solomon (Eds.), *The healing power of emotion: Affective neuroscience, development, and clinical practice* (pp. 112–144). W.W. Norton & Company.

Schore, A. (2019). *Right-brain psychotherapy.* W.W. Norton & Company.

Skean, K. R. (2018). AEDP and cultural competence in developmental trauma treatment. *Pragmatic Case Studies in Psychotherapy, 14*(1), 69–76. https://doi.org/10.14713/pcsp.v14i1.2034

Squire, L. R. (2004). Memory systems of the brain: A brief history and current perspective. *Neurobiology of Learning and Memory, 82*(3), 171–177. https://doi.org/10.1016/j.nlm.2004.06.005

Stiles, W. B., Honos-Webb, L., & Surko, M. (1998) Responsiveness in psychotherapy. *Clinical Psychology: Science and Practice, 5*(4), 439–458. https://doi.org/10.1111/j.1468-2850.1998.tb00166.x

Stiles, W. B., & Horvath, A. O. (2017). Appropriate responsiveness as a contribution to therapist effects. In L. G. Castonguay & C. E. Hill (Eds.), *How and why are some therapists better than others? Understanding therapist effects* (pp. 71–84). American Psychological Association. https://doi.org/10.1037/0000034-005

Taylor, J. M., & Neimeyer, G. J. (2017). Lifelong professional improvement: The evolution of continuing education. In T. G. Rousmaniere, R. Goodyear, S. D. Miller, & B. Wampold (Eds.), *The cycle of excellence: Using deliberate practice to improve supervision and training* (pp. 219–248). Wiley Blackwell.

Tracey, T. J. G., Wampold, B. E., Goodyear, R. K., & Lichtenberg, J. W. (2015). Improving expertise in psychotherapy. *Psychotherapy Bulletin, 50*(1), 7–13.

Tronick, E. Z. (1998). Dyadically expanded states of consciousness and the process of therapeutic change. *Infant Mental Health Journal, 19*(3), 290–299. https://doi.org/10.1002/(SICI)1097-0355(199823)19:3<290::AID-IMHJ4>3.0.CO;2-Q

Tunnell, G., & Osiason, J. (2021). Historical context: AEDP's place in the world of psychotherapy. In D. Fosha (Ed.), *Undoing aloneness and the transformation of suffering into flourishing: AEDP 2.0* (pp. 83–106). American Psychological Association. https://doi.org/10.1037/0000232-004

Wallin, D. (2007). *Attachment in psychotherapy*. Guilford Press.

Wass, R., & Golding, C. (2014). Sharpening a tool for teaching: The zone of proximal development. *Teaching in Higher Education, 19*(6), 671–684. https://doi.org/10.1080/13562517.2014.901958

Yeung, D. (2021). What went right? What happens in the brain during AEDP's metatherapeutic processing. In D. Fosha (Ed.), *Undoing aloneness and the transformation of suffering into flourishing: AEDP 2.0* (pp. 349–376). American Psychological Association. https://doi.org/10.1037/0000232-014

Zaretskii, V. (2009). The zone of proximal development: What Vygotsky did not have time to write. *Journal of Russian & East European Psychology, 47*(6), 70–93. https://doi.org/10.2753/RPO1061-0405470604

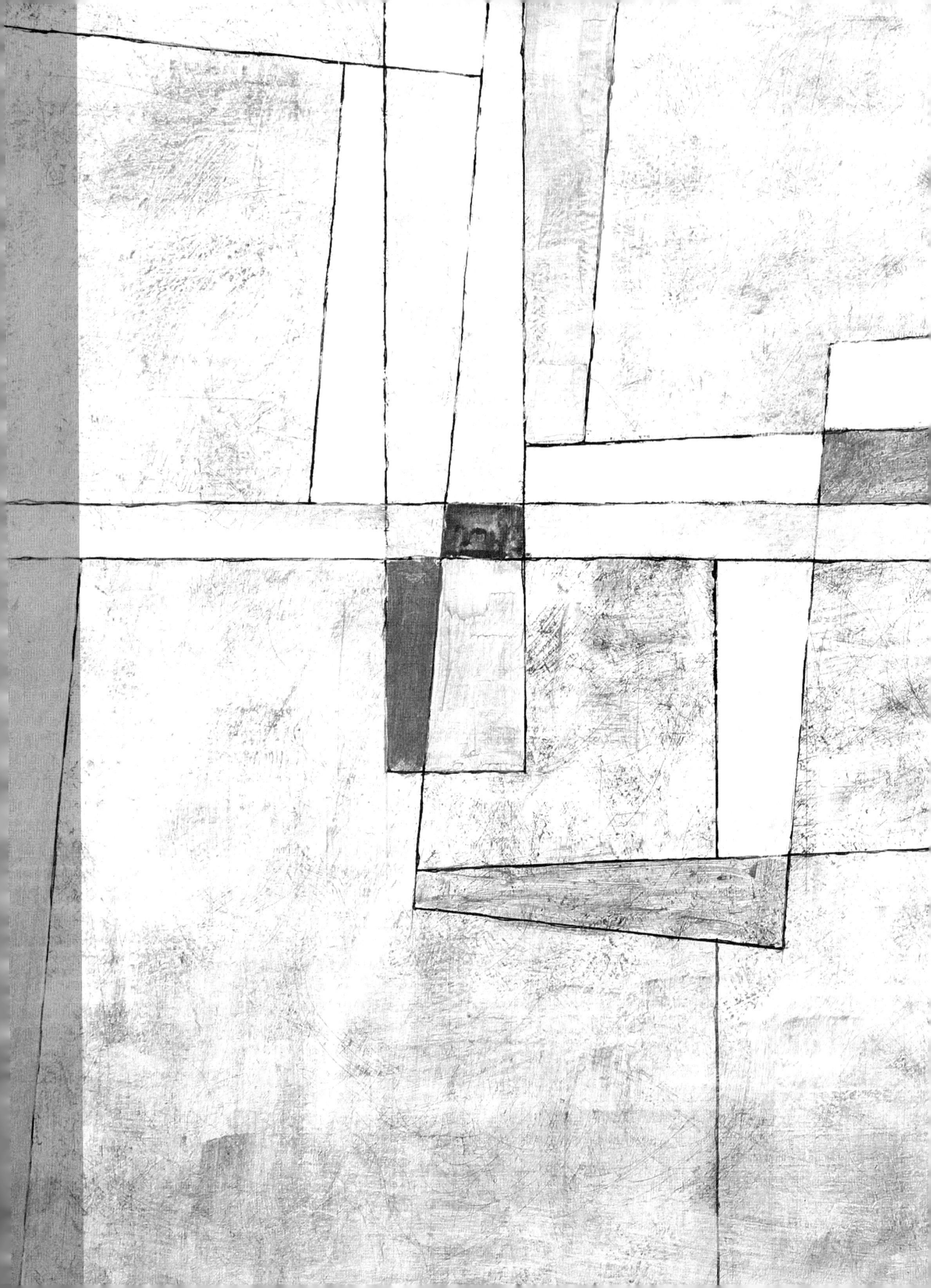

Index

A

Accelerated experiential dynamic psychotherapy (AEDP)
  overview of, 9–10
  research on, 11–12
Active effort, 209
AEDP Essential Skills Course, 16
AEDP Fidelity Scale, 4, 12, 16
AEDP Immersion Course, 16
AEDP Institute, 3, 12
Affective-relational patterns, 74
Affirmative work with defenses, 14, 119–128
  client statements, 123–125
  helpful hint, 120
  instructions, 122
  skill criteria, 120
  skill description, 119–120
  therapist examples, 120–121
  therapist responses, 126–128
Affirming, 13, 63–71
  client statements, 66–68
  instructions, 65
  skill criteria, 64
  skill description, 63–64
  therapist examples, 64
  therapist responses, 69–71
Alliance, trainee–trainer, 212
Aloneness. See Undoing aloneness
Anxiety, working with, 14, 107–116, 194–196
  client statements, 111–113
  instructions, 110
  skill criterion, 108
  skill description, 107–108
  therapist examples, 108–109
  therapist responses, 114–116
  in triangle of experience, 10
Appropriate responsiveness, 191, 204
Attachment relationships, 9–10
Attunement, 15

B

Behaviors
  celebration of healthy, 144
  nonverbal. See Nonverbal behaviors

Body posture, 15
Breaks, 210

C

Challenge, level of. See Level of challenge
Change for the better, experience of, 157
Client outcomes, 211
Coker, Jerry, 8
Complex reactions, toward the trainer, 212
Conceição, N., 224
Consciousness, dyadic states of, 74
Core states, 10
Customization of exercises, 202–203
Cycle of deliberate practice, 7

D

Davis, Miles, 8
Declarative knowledge, 8–9
Defenses, 10. See also Affirmative work with defenses
Deliberate practice diary form, 219–220
Depression, 194
Difficulty assessments and adjustments, 192–194, 203–205,
    207–208, 215–217. See also Zone of proximal development
Discussion, of exercises, 21
Dissatisfaction, 196
Driving analogy, 12
Dyadic states of consciousness, 74

E

Eating disorders, 195
Effort, flow vs., 209
Emotional stimuli, realistic, 201–202
Emotions, 11, 131
Empathy, 85
Ericsson, K. Anders, 7
Evaluations, final, 21
Exercises
  customization of, 202–203
  reviews of, 21
Experiences, 10, 157

Exploring and staying with physical experience, 13, 37–51
    dialogues, 40–45
    instructions, 39
    skill criteria, 38
    skill description, 37–38
    therapist examples, 38
    therapist responses, 46–51

F

Facial expressions, 15
Feedback, for exercises, 21, 206–207
Feelings, in triangle of experience, 10
Final evaluations, 21
Flow, effort vs., 209
Fosha, D., 12, 16, 224
Four-state model, 10

G

Geller, S., 15
Gladwell, Malcolm, 7
Gleiser, K., 224
Greenberg, L. S., 73
Guy, J. D., 213

H

Halliday, K., 15, 143, 224
Hanakawa, Y., 224, 227
Harrison, R., 224
Healthy behavior, celebration of, 144
Hendel, H. 224, 227, 228

I

Improvisation, 8
Improvised task performance, 9
Initiating portrayals, 14, 131–140
    client statements, 135–137
    helpful hint, 132
    instructions, 134
    skill criteria, 132
    skill description, 131–132
    therapist examples, 132–133
    therapist responses, 138–140
Insomnia, 195, 196
Instability, of relationships, 196
Internal and somatic experiences, 157
Isolation, 195
Iwakabe, S., 11, 224

J

Jazz analogy, 8, 191, 203

K

Knowledge, declarative vs. procedural, 8–9
Kranz, K., 224

L

Lability, of mood, 196
Lamagna, J., 15, 224, 228
Learning, state-dependent, 8
Learning processes, 202
Level of challenge, 192–194, 202–203, 215–217
Levenson, H., 4, 12, 227
Lipton, B., 15, 224
Loneliness, 195. *See also* Undoing aloneness

M

Mastery learning, simulation-based, 8
Medley, B., 224
Metaprocessing, 14, 95–104
    client statements, 99–101
    instructions, 98
    and self-disclosure, 86
    skill criteria, 96
    skill description, 95–96
    therapist examples, 97
    therapist responses, 102–104
Metatherapeutic processing, 10, 15, 157–180
    dialogues, 161–170
    helpful hint, 159
    instructions, 160
    skill criteria, 159
    skill description, 157–158
    therapist example, 159
    therapist responses, 171–180
Mindfulness, 205
Mock sessions, 191–196
    client profiles, 194–196
    overview, 191–192
    procedure, 192–193
    varying the level of challenge, 193–194
Moment-to-moment tracking, 12–13, 25–34
    client statements, 29–31
    helpful hints, 26
    instructions, 28
    skill criterion, 26
    skill description, 25–26
    therapist examples, 26–27
    therapist responses, 32–34
Monitoring of training results, 211
Mood lability, 196
Multicultural, 225–226

N

Nonsuicidal self-harm, 196
Nonverbal behaviors, 15, 21, 54, 64, 193
Norcross, J. C., 213
Notsu, H., 11

O

Orlinsky, D. E., 213
Outcomes, client, 211
Outliers (Gladwell), 7

P

Pando-Mars, K., 224
Panic attack, 195
Paraverbal behaviors, 54
Physical experience. *See* Exploring and staying with physical experience
Playfulness, 210
Portrayals. *See* Initiating portrayals
Positive emotions, 11
Practice session transcript, 183–188
Prenn, N. C. N., 3, 205, 224
Presence with trainee, trainers', 54
Privileging transformation strivings, 14–15, 143–154
    client statements, 147–149
    helpful hint, 144

instructions, 146
    skill criteria, 144
    skill description, 143–144
    therapist examples, 144–145
    therapist responses, 150–154
Procedural knowledge, 9
Proximal development, zone of, 207–209

R

Reactions toward the trainer, trainees', 212
Real clients, trainee performance with, 208
Realistic emotional stimuli, 201–202
Reassurance, need for, 195
Rehearsal, 203
Relational experiences, 10, 157
Relational experiences, core, 10
Relationship instability, 196
Relationships, attachment, 9–10
Repetition, of an activity, 9
Responsiveness, appropriate, 191, 204
Reviews, of exercises, 21
Role-playing, 131, 201–202
Ronnestad, M. H., 213
Russell, E., 15, 108

S

"Saying all of it," 73
Self-disclosure. *See* Self-involving self-disclosure; Self-revealing
    self-disclosure
Self-efficacy, 205
Self-harm, 196
Self-involving self-disclosure, 13, 73–82
    client statements, 77–79
    instructions, 76
    skill criteria, 74
    skill description, 73–74
    therapist examples, 75
    therapist responses, 80–82
Self-revealing self-disclosure, 13, 85–93
    client statements, 88–90
    helpful hints, 86
    instructions, 87
    skill criterion, 86
    skill description, 85–86
    therapist examples, 86
    therapist responses, 91–93
Shame, 195
Simulation-based mastery learning, 8
Skill criteria, 20–21
State-dependent learning, 8
States, core, 10
Strivings, transformative. *See* Privileging transformation strivings
Suicide, 90
Syllabus, with embedded examples, 223

T

Teaching styles, 202
10,000-hour rule, 7
Therapeutic alliance, working, 11
Thoma, N., 224
Trainee(s)
    guidance for, 208–213
    own therapy, 212–213
    own training process, 209–210, 212
    performance with real clients of, 208
    personal development of, 212
    privacy of, 206
    questions for, 213
    reactions toward the trainer of, 212
    and responsive treatment, 204–205
    self-evaluation by, 206–208
    trainers' presence with, 54
    well-being of, 205
    work as therapists of, 212
    work performance of, 206–207
Trainee–trainer alliance, 212
Trainer(s)
    and being present with trainees, 54
    guidance for, 201–213
    and responsive treatment, 204–205
    role of, 20
    self-evaluations of, 206
    trainees' reactions toward, 212
Transcript, of practice session, 183–188
Transformative strivings. *See* Privileging transformation strivings
Triangle of experience, 10

U

Undoing aloneness, 12–13, 53–61
    client statements, 56–58
    instructions, 55
    skill criteria, 54
    skill description, 53–54
    therapist examples, 54
    therapist responses, 59–61
Unfinished business, 131
Unprocessed emotions, 131

V

Voice quality and tone, 15, 54, 183, 193
Vulnerability, of therapists, 74

W

Watson, J. C., 73
Working therapeutic alliance, 11

Y

Yeung, D., 224

Z

Zone of proximal development, 207–209

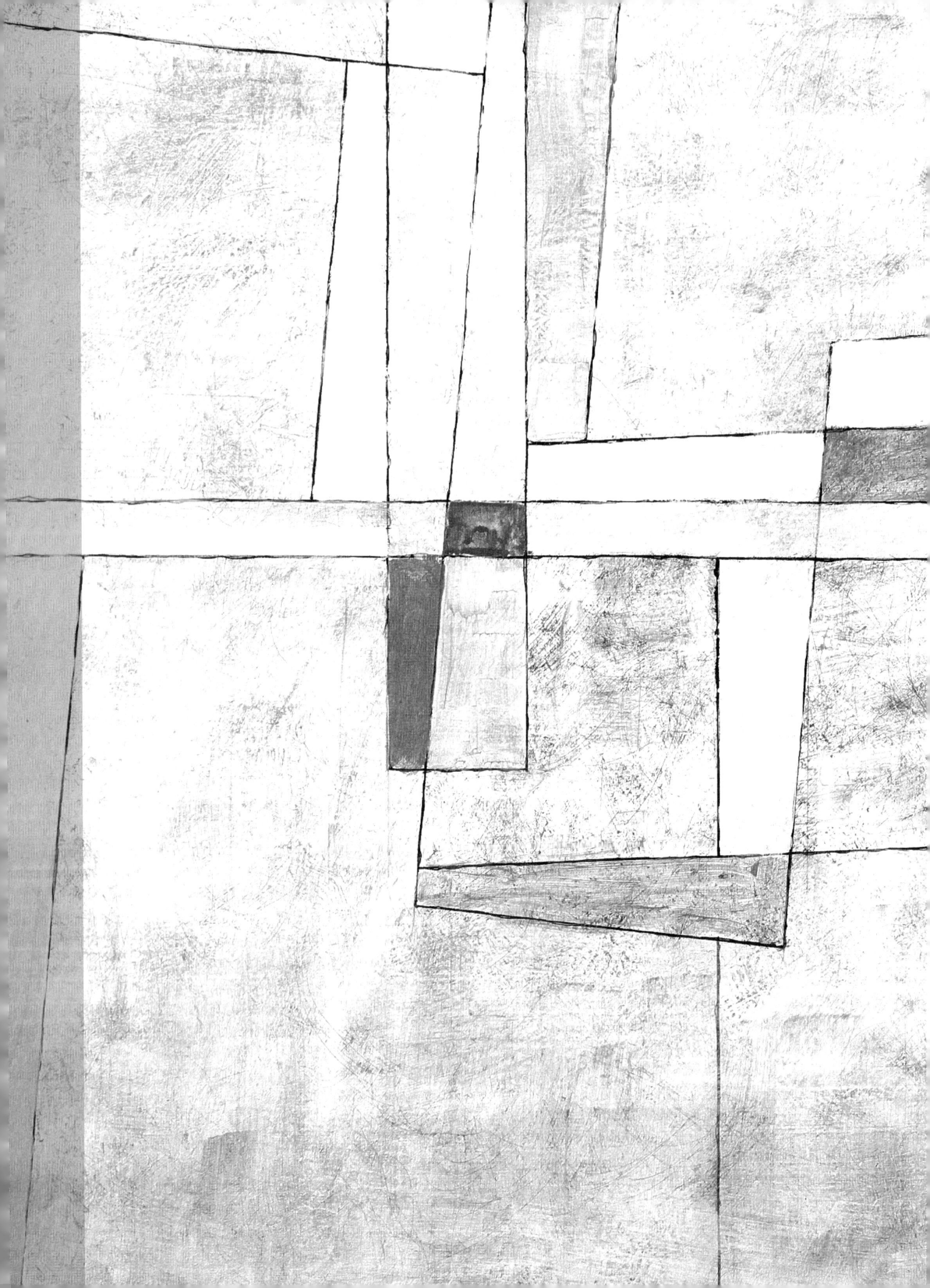

About the Authors

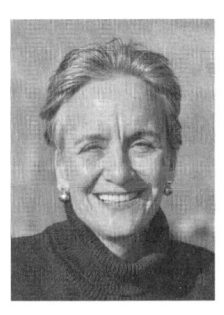

Natasha C. N. Prenn, LCSW, is senior faculty at the AEDP Institute. She sees individuals and couples for therapy and clinicians for accelerated experiential dynamic psychotherapy (AEDP) supervision. She pioneered the AEDP Essential Skills and Advanced Skills Courses. She is coauthor, with Diana Fosha, of a book in the American Psychological Association's (APA's) Clinical Supervision Essentials series (edited by Hanna Levenson and Arpana G. Inman): *Supervision Essentials for Accelerated Experiential Dynamic Psychotherapy*. Prenn is a founding editor of *Transformance: The AEDP Journal*. She has presented numerous workshops and trainings and written several book chapters and articles focused on the nuts and bolts of what to actually say and do in AEDP psychotherapy sessions.

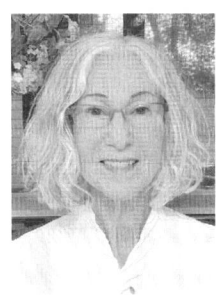

Hanna Levenson, PhD, is professor emerita at the Wright Institute in Berkeley, California. She sees individuals and couples for therapy and professionals for consultation, in addition to her writing and research. For 20 years Dr. Levenson was clinical professor in the Department of Psychiatry, University of California School of Medicine and director of the Brief Therapy Program at the Veterans Administration Medical Center. She has been specializing in the areas of brief, experiential-relational-dynamic psychotherapy for individuals and couples, and clinical supervision for almost 50 years. She is the author of over 80 professional papers and six books, most recently *Deliberate Practice in Psychodynamic Psychotherapy* (APA, 2023) and *Deliberate Practice in Emotionally Focused Couple Therapy* (APA, 2025). In addition, she has six professionally produced videos of her clinical work. Dr. Levenson is the recipient of the Distinguished Contribution to Psychology as a Profession Award given by the California Psychological Association, and the Certificate of Recognition Award from the National Organization of Veterans Administration Psychologists.

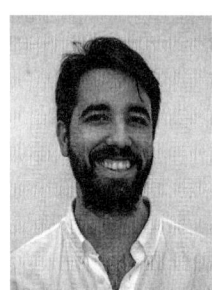

Alexandre Vaz, PhD, is cofounder and chief academic officer of Sentio University and the Sentio Counseling Center. He provides workshops, webinars, and advanced clinical training and supervision to clinicians around the world. Dr. Vaz is the author/coeditor of many books on deliberate practice and psychotherapy training. He has held multiple committee roles for the Society for the Exploration of Psychotherapy Integration (SEPI) and the Society for Psychotherapy Research (SPR). Dr. Vaz is founder and host of "Psychotherapy Expert Talks," an acclaimed interview series with distinguished psychotherapists and therapy researchers.

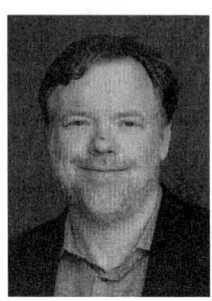

Tony Rousmaniere, PsyD, is cofounder and program director of Sentio University and the Sentio Counseling Center. He provides workshops, webinars, and advanced clinical training and supervision to clinicians around the world. Dr. Rousmaniere is the author/coeditor of many books on deliberate practice and psychotherapy training. In 2017 he published the widely cited article "What Your Therapist Doesn't Know" in *The Atlantic*. Dr. Rousmaniere supports the open-data movement and publishes his aggregated clinical outcome data, in deidentified form, on his website at https://drtonyr.com/. Dr. Rousmaniere is president of Division 29 of the American Psychological Association (Society for the Advancement of Psychotherapy).